Heaven Scent

Christine Stalsonburg

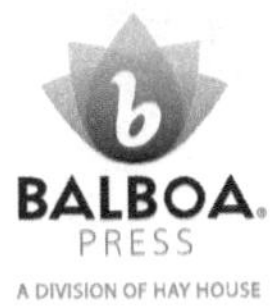

BALBOA. PRESS

A DIVISION OF HAY HOUSE

Balboa Press books may be ordered through booksellers or by contacting:

Balboa Press
A Division of Hay House
1663 Liberty Drive
Bloomington, IN 47403
www.balboapress.com
1 (877) 407-4847

Print information available on the last page.

ISBN: 978-1-9822-1424-1 (sc)
ISBN: 978-1-9822-1426-5 (hc)
ISBN: 978-1-9822-1425-8 (e)

Library of Congress Control Number: 2018912282

Balboa Press rev. date: 10/17/2018

Contents

Introduction

Essential oils have been a part of my way of life for many years. When I first started using essential oils, there was little information out there on the safe and effective way to use them. After spending hours trying to find a reference book that I could use that would be simple, accurate, and safe, I decided to write one of my own.

Years of education and research have gone into developing what I hope will be your go-to guide when you have questions about essential oils or are looking for a safe recipe to help support your body.

As a licensed massage therapist, a certified clinical aromatherapist, and the founder of Angelic Energy Mind, Body, Spirit, I have developed dozens of custom blends that have helped hundreds of clients with both physical and emotional issues they were experiencing.

Essential oils are not meant to be a replacement for medical advice or treatments. They are here to help support healthy balance in your mind, body, and spirit.

It is my wish that you will come to love and respect these precious oils just as much as I have and that you will grow to have a new appreciation and respect for the amazing therapeutic properties they have to offer.

Heaven Scent brings you thirty-six of my most favorite essential oils. Several of them are extremely rare and for this reason are used in my recipes sparingly. My reason for this is so that, as an industry, we do not cause an over harvest of these resources that is not sustainable. God has provided us with these amazing plants, trees, and flowers to assist us in healing ourselves. It is our duty to honor these gifts and use them wisely for their intended purpose.

The information in this book is for educational purposes. This information has not been evaluated by the Food and Drug Administration. This information is not intended to diagnose, treat, cure, or prevent any disease.

May you be blessed with a sense of peace and serenity as you sit with *Heaven Scent* and enjoy your journey through some amazing essential oils.

History of Essential Oils and How They Support Your Body

The History of Essential Oils

In ancient times, essential oils were used in aromatherapy to aid people with their physical and emotional health. In the past, they have been used by many people all over the world and in different cultures to do this. The history of essential oils is a long one. Thousands of years ago, the Chinese used plants with aromatic qualities for healing. Although these plant substances were used in the medical practices of the day, they had not yet been distilled into essential oils.

The Egyptians, and perhaps also the Persians and the people of India, were the first to make distillation machines. Oil of cedarwood, distilled with such machines, was used along with myrrh, cinnamon, clove, and nutmeg oils to embalm the dead.

The Egyptians were concerned more with the sense of smell than with any of the other senses. They believed that it was the most important and dominant sense. They incorporated the essential oils they made into their medicine, cosmetics, and fragrances.

The use of essential oils was taken up by the Greeks next. Hippocrates did an ancient form of aromatherapy. A Greek named Megalleon invented a perfume called megalleon. This substance was used in aromatherapy and as an anti-inflammatory essential oil to heal wounds. A Roman named Discorides wrote on the uses of over five hundred different plant substances and distillations that were made of many of them. However, these distillations didn't produce essential oils. Instead, they made floral-smelling waters.

Avicenna was a Persian philosopher-scientist who refined the process by inventing a distillation machine with a coiled cooling pipe. This allowed for more effective cooling. Eventually, the focus shifted toward an emphasis on true essential oils and their therapeutic uses.

Paracelcus was a fifteenth-century doctor who began using the term *essence*. His emphasis was using essential oils for medicine. During this time, many new essential oils were being produced. Among them were juniper, rosemary, rose, and sage. During the sixteenth century, people would go to their apothecary to get essential oils for many different uses. Around this time, the advent of new essential oils flourished. In the next few centuries, essential oils changed little except in their use in perfumes.

In the twentieth century, the major chemical ingredients of essential oils were identified. Scientists started becoming more interested in the subject of essential oils, which became a problem for those interested in the use of true essential oils.

Much of twentieth-century science had been consumed with creating synthetic versions of essential oils. However, an early twentieth-century Frenchman named Gattefosse became increasingly involved with the study of essential oils and their medicinal values. He was the first to use the term *aromatherapy*. Aromatherapy and the use of essential oils was not well known in English-speaking countries. Robert B. Tisserand changed all that. He wrote the first English book on the subject, along with many other books and articles.

As the years went by, people were becoming more and more interested in natural ways of doing things. They wanted to find ways to soothe their minds and comfort their bodies without synthetic drugs. Essential oils gave them a way to do it.

Historically, there has not been significant evidence-based research done on humans. Most of the evidence-based research has been done on animals, and some has been done internally at very high doses. It is important to keep this in mind when you are looking at essential oils to support your well-being. Just because something works well or causes issues in an animal does not mean we will see the exact same results with humans. It is for this reason that we use this research as a guide to taking a safe approach when using essential oils. Western cultures have been somewhat resistant to using essential oils as complementary medicine but are starting to become more open to the benefits that come from their use. More and more studies are being conducted and will most likely continue over the years. Canada, Australia, and many European countries have used essential oils in their medical treatments of patients for many years with some powerful outcomes. Currently, in the United States, the FDA has not evaluated or approved any essential oils for treating or curing any medical issues. It is vital that you remember that essential oils are not a cure or quick fix for anything, but they can help support your body in its natural healing process back to a state of well-being.

How Do Essential Oils Work to Support Our Bodies?

To have a more complete idea of how essential oils work in your body, you need an understanding of how your body works to support itself on a daily basis. The body is a complex system comprised of cells, tissues, organs, systems, and organisms. This book is not designed to be an anatomy and physiology lesson, so I aim to keep things simple as they relate to essential oils.

The cell is the smallest living unit in our bodies and also the basic unit of life. Cellular health is vitally important to the overall well-being of every human. Cells of similar composition join together to make either areolar, adipose, or fibrous tissue. Tissue joins together and then becomes an organ, such as a kidney and liver. These organs make up different systems in our body, including skeletal, nervous, circulatory, respiratory, digestive, and muscular. Our organs interact with each other to maintain a balance in our body, which is called homeostasis. These systems make up the organism that we call the human body.

The human body is made up of various chemicals. We do not think of our bodies as housing for chemicals, but in essence, that is exactly what it is. Three main chemicals that make up our bodies are oxygen at 65 percent, hydrogen at 18 percent, and nitrogen at almost 10 percent (these percentages are by mass, not by fraction of atoms).

Now, let's fast-forward and look at what makes up essential oils. Essential oils are made up of chemicals, primarily carbon, hydrogen, oxygen, and sometimes nitrogen and sulfur. How these chemicals bond together will determine what the chemical family or constituents will be. It is the chemical constituents that provide the therapeutic properties of the essential oil. Let's take a look at nine of the most common chemical families within an essential oil to determine what areas of the body it may be best suited to support. These chemical families are monoterpenes, sesquiterpenes, monoterpennols, sesquiterpenols, esthers, aldehydes, phenols, ketones, oxides, and esters. Within each of these chemical families, there are chemical components or constituents that further define the possible therapeutic properties of the oil. To determine the best essential oil to help support the body, you will need to examine the specific chemical components of the oil, not just the chemical family. This section is not intended to be a chemistry lesson, just a brief overview to introduce you to the science behind why essential oils work in supporting our bodies. Understanding the chemical families a bit better will help you when you are looking at possible safety concerns with individual oils. When I look at the gas chromatography/mass spectrometry (GC/MS) chemical testing sheets, I look for significant percentages of these constituents when choosing which oil will be best for a particular situation. It is not an exact science, and much depends on my experience with a particular oil and the research I have found.

The first two we will take a look at come from the terpene family. A terpene molecule contains only carbon and hydrogen. Having no oxygen in these particular oils makes them volatile and susceptible to oxidization. Due to the size of these molecules, they can pass through the blood-brain barrier and be directly absorbed into the brain tissue.

Monoterpenes, in general, are known to have therapeutic properties of an antiseptic, antibacterial, and mild analgesic. In general, they have a stimulating effect and can soothe irritated tissues.

Sesquiterpenes, in general, are known to have therapeutic properties of an anti-inflammatory, antispasmodic, and antiseptic. Typically they have strong aromas. Oils in this category each have specific therapeutic effects and should be looked at on a more individual basis rather than as a broad category.

Monoterpenols, in general, have significant anti-infectious properties. They are also known for being gentle to the skin and mucous membranes (with the exception of peppermint). Long-term use can show helpful results as immune stimulants.

Sesquiterpenols, in general, have varied properties of grounding, sedative, and immune-stimulating effects. They are generally safe and gentle on the skin when diluted appropriately.

Oxides, in general, are beneficial due to the 1.8 cineole they contain. Note that not all oxides contain this chemical component. It is this 1.8 cineole that gives them their camphor aroma and gives them strong antiviral, antibacterial, and expectorant properties. Essential oils high in 1.8 cineole are contraindicated in use with children under the age of ten.

Esthers, in general, are known to have therapeutic properties of being relaxing, calming, and balancing to the body.

Aldehydes, in general, are known to have therapeutic properties of being anti-infectious and anti-inflammatory and can be calming to the central nervous system. Word of caution: These oils are skin irritating and should be used in low dilution rates (1 percent if using on the skin) to avoid adverse reactions. If you have sensitive skin to begin with, you will definitely want to do skin patch testing before using it on the body in general application.

Ketones, in general, are known to have therapeutic properties of supporting respiratory issues and assisting with wound healing. Safety concerns vary with ketones, so be sure to not generalize this chemical family.

Phenols, in general, are known to be irritating to the skin and mucous membranes. Just as we saw with aldehydes, these oils should be diluted to no more than a 1 percent solution when using on the skin and should be used with skin-nourishing oils to complement the blend. These oil types tend to have very powerful antibacterial and antiseptic properties but should not be used for long periods of time.

An important thing to remember when blending essential oils is that not always will blending two oils with the same therapeutic properties cause the blend to have synergistic values. Blending of essential oils is a very complex art that requires research of the blending capabilities of the oils you are using. There are occasions when blending two essential oils with the same therapeutic properties will result in an antagonistic or negative effect. It is similar to taking two types of prescription pain medications. The outcome may not necessarily be more pain relief and in some cases could cause harm.

How Do Essential Oils Get into Your System?

Essential oils can be introduced into the body through injection, inhalation, ingestion, and dermal absorption. I will be address inhalation and dermal absorption in this book. Injection and ingestion should always be reserved for use only under the supervision of a licensed healthcare provider who specializes in the area of essential oil, as these methods can be extremely dangerous.

Inhalation of essential oils has great benefit for quick response by the body. Our bodies are equipped with a filtering system in our brain, called the blood-brain barrier. This filtering system prevents potential damaging substances from directly reaching the brain and spinal fluid due to the very small size of molecules that can pass through this barrier. The chemical component, sesquiterpene, is small enough to successfully cross the blood-brain barrier. Many essential oils are high in this chemical component and when inhaled will have an almost immediate brain response to the therapeutic properties of the essential oil.

Essential oils not containing sesquiterpenes will still have great benefit through inhalation, just not by crossing the blood-brain barrier. In these such cases, the essential oils will be absorbed through the bloodstream through the lungs.

Dermal absorption can affect the body in one of two ways: it can have a local effect, or it can have a systemic effect. When we apply a lotion or carrier oil mixed with essential oils to our skin, it will be absorbed into the dermal cells of the skin. There is a barrier between the surface of the skin and the circulatory system beneath the skin. This barrier is called the stratum corneum. Some essential oils can penetrate the stratum corneum and enter the bloodstream, causing systemic therapeutic effects on the body. When the chemical components cannot penetrate the stratum corneum, the essential oil will only have localized therapeutic effects on the body, which will be isolated to the area of application.

Once an essential oil enters the bloodstream, it needs to find a manner in which to circulate through the bloodstream. Since the majority of the makeup of our blood is water based and essential oils do not mix with water, they need to find a protein to bind to in order to distribute therapeutic properties systemically.

From Seed to Bottle

In this chapter, I will take you through the process of growing, harvesting, processing, extracting, and bottling essential oils. There are hundreds of farmers around the world who grow, harvest, and distill for essential oil companies. The process before the essential oil gets into the bottle is just as important, if not more important, than the bottling itself. The information you will learn will empower you to be a better consumer when you are shopping for essential oils. You come away with a better understanding of how these precious essential oils get from the fields to your hands.

Growing Process

Plants grown for the production of essential oils should always be grown in their indigenous climate. Have you ever tried to grow a cactus in northern Michigan? The answer is, probably not. There are many reasons why the cactus would not thrive: improper soil, fluctuating temperatures, and lack of sufficient sunshine are just a few. You would have to build an environment that would duplicate the desert for the cactus to even survive. Chances are it might never bloom, and if it did, it might produce fewer flowers with less brilliant colors. I give you this example because this is the exact same thing that happens when you try to grow plants, trees, and shrubs for essential oil use in environments where they are not indigenous.

When plants are grown in their indigenous environment, they thrive on the nutrient-rich soil native to the area and rarely have to deal with insects attacking them. Temperature ranges are best suited for them, as well as appropriate sunlight. When plants are given these surroundings to grow in, they will develop into wonderful sources for essential oil extraction. When a plant has to deal with stressors on its system, like harsh temperatures or pesticides, it causes the plant to not be as rich in essential oils. We will not see this until the plant is harvested and the appropriate plant part has been distilled and tested for its chemical components.

Harvesting and Processing

Essential oils are derived from a variety of different parts of a plant, such as seeds, bark, leaves, stems, roots, flowers, fruit, resin, etc. This information is important when we speak about the chemical components of an essential oil. Let's use lavender as an example. The only part of the lavender plant that should be used for essential oil distillation are the flowers. It takes a tremendous amount of flowers to make a drop of essential oil.

- It takes three pounds of lavender to make fifteen milliliters of essential oil.
- It takes two hundred fifty thousand rose petals to make five milliliters of essential oil.
- It takes fifteen lemons to make fifteen milliliters of essential oil.

You can see just how precious these essential oils are and how much plant material it takes to distill the oils. It is for this reason that the cost of unadulterated essential oils can be high.

Plants at the time of harvest are living organisms. Everything that is done to the plant from the point of harvest through distillation damages or breaks down the plant parts, which can cause the chemical component values to change. Plant parts should be handled gently, so as not to start the oxidation process, which will cause damage.

Extraction

There are several methods to extract the essential oils from the plant parts, including cold distillation, steam distillation, cold press, and solvent extraction. The method used will affect the chemical components in the essential oil as well as shelf life and safety concerns. It is important to always know how your essential oils were extracted.

The cold distillation process is not frequently done but has amazing benefits to the essential oil. When this process is used, the plant part has much less damage done to it versus using steam to extract the oils. The entire process can take up to ninety days (typical steam distillation can be done in a little over an hour). One can see how this process is not suited for mass producers of essential oils. Time to bottle is prohibitive for them. By using this method, we tend to see an essential oil that virtually has an eternal shelf life because it doesn't cause the massive oxidation that happens with steam distillation. There is an amazing distillery on the island of Maui, Scent of Knowing, that uses this process and produces some incredible essential oils. I had the honor to visit this distillery and meet all of his wonderful essential oils, some of which were over twenty years old and had the most fragrant aromas. The distiller attributes the longevity of the shelf life to the cold distillation process that he uses.

Steam distillation is the most common of the extraction methods used for essential oils. A combination of steam and pressure passes through the plant material, releasing the oils from the plant. It is an extremely quick process where mass quantities of essential oils can be produced in relatively short periods of time. The volatile components are then separated from the water used for the distillation.

The oil is bottled for essential oil sale, and the remaining water is bottled as a hydrosol. Hydrosols have many wonderful uses, especially for children. The potency of the hydrosol is much less than an essential oil, and therefore it is very safe for direct use on children of any age as well as for undiluted use on the skin. It is important to remember that citrus essential oils that are extracted using this process are not phytotoxic and are safe to use diluted on the skin when going out into direct sunlight.

Cold press extraction is typically used with citrus oils such as grapefruits, limes, lemons, bergamots, sweet oranges, tangerines, and mandarin oranges. Over the decades, it has become much more efficient to process with the use of mechanical pressing. During the process, the rind of the fruit is punctured with spikes to allow the release of the oils when the fruit is spun mechanically. The centrifugal force separates the fruit juice from the oil. This method leave small amounts of nonvolatile residue in the oil, giving it an aroma that is very closely matched with the fresh fruit peel. The disadvantage to this process is that these same residues can cause diffusers to clog and stain fabric, and it results in shorter shelf lives. Essential oils that are cold pressed will also be photo-toxic.

Solvent extraction is typically used on very delicate plants flowers such as rose and jasmine. This is a two-step process where the plant part is either gently broken apart to allow for the solvent (usually an alcohol-based solvent) or the solvent and plant part are placed in a spinning drum to extract the essential oils and fragrance. The mixture is now vacuum distilled to ensure that any excessive solvent is removed. This process is repeated a second time. The final product of this extraction process is referred to as an absolute and not an actual essential oil. Absolutes are commonly used in the perfume industry due to the absolute being a very aroma-rich product.

Where to Purchase Your Oils and Who to Get Guidance From

In recent years, essential oils have become one of the country's most talked about products. There are many outlets to purchase them, and there are literally thousands of people who claim to have knowledge about essential oils who are giving guidance on how they can support your body. In the sections below, I will discuss how to make an educated choice in where to purchase your essential oils and who to get your guidance from.

In the United States, there are no regulations on the sale and use of essential oils. Essential oils are not a treatment or cure for anything, so they are not regulated by the FDA. This is a double-edged sword and is the root of much confusion for the consumer who is seeking essential oils to use. Eastern medicine has been using essential oils for hundreds of years with great success. Western medicine is barely scratching the surface on embracing the incredible therapeutic benefits of essential oils. We are just starting to see testing and exploration of essential oils as a holistic approach to illness and disease. Many of the state-licensed holistic and herbalists practitioners have studied the therapeutic benefits of essential oils and use them in their practices. Midlevel and unlicensed practitioners, called certified aromatherapists, also use essential oils to assist their clients in alternative ways to support their bodies. This is where the confusion starts for consumers. If consumers embrace a natural approach to their lifestyle and want to learn more about the benefits of essential oils but does not want to enlist the services of a licensed practitioner, they will turn to the other outlets for the sale of essential oils: health food stores, drug stores, grocery stores, multilevel marketing companies, apothecary shops, just to name a few. There are two important areas to explore. Where do I purchase my essential oils, and who do I seek out for guidance on how to safely use them?

If you remember in the last chapter, I took you through the growing, harvesting, and processing process. You might have been wondering why I went down that road. There was a method to my madness. I wanted you to see the steps of the process so you could better understand how these steps play a vital part in the quality of the essential oils that are available for purchase. Essential oils are at their maximum therapeutic benefit when they are grown in their natural habitat, in perfect climate conditions, with no pesticides or fertilizers. Plants use their oils to protect themselves from harsh growing conditions and other inorganic chemicals placed on them. If a plant has to use the lion's share of its protective oils fighting off the elements, it dilutes the precious chemical components that give it its therapeutic benefit. With this in mind, you will always want to know the origin of the essential oil (what country was it grown in), and you will want to know the quality of the oil.

Let's bust a myth. There is no such thing as a "therapeutic-grade" essential oil. Again, no one regulates this industry, and therefore there is no standard for this catchphrase that a few larger essential oil sales companies have chosen to place on the essential oils they are selling. The *only* way to define the true quality of an essential oil is with third-party testing through GC/MS (gas chromatography/mass spectrometry). This testing breaks down the oil and reports every single chemical component that is in the essential oil and will show if there are any contaminants in the essential oil. You always want to make sure that this testing is done by a third party and not the distiller or the bottling company. Why, you ask? Good question. The answer is adulteration. Adulteration is where either an odorous or non-odorous substance is added in an attempt to dilute the essential oil to increase profit margins. You cannot tell by smell alone the quality of the oils. Many essential oils are quite costly because of how much plant material is needed to obtain the precious oils, and some distillers and/or bottling companies are looking for ways to maximize their profits. With the industry not being regulated for quality, they can certainly do and claim anything they want to, and the consumer typically never knows unless they ask for these test results or consults with a practitioner who is knowledgeable in this area and knows what to look for and ask for when recommending essential oils for you to use. Having the distiller or bottling company do their own testing is a slippery slope and leaves much temptation on the table for adulteration.

Now that you know what to look for in essential oil quality, how do you choose someone to guide you through the safe use of essential oils? Again, this is an unregulated field in the United States. The first course of action is to establish care with a licensed holistic practitioner for your guidance. Like any other professional, this can be a costly endeavor that many do not have the disposable income for and is usually not covered under most health insurance plans. A certified aromatherapist is the next best choice. Aromatherapists, as well as anyone who says they have been through a certified program for essential oils, are not governed by any regulating agency in the United States. The differences in the degrees of training are jaw dropping. It can vary from eight hours of training to over one thousand hours of training for certification programs. It is critically important that you ask what type of training someone has before you heed their advice and guidance on something that will have a huge impact on your body.

Just like the research you did on the company to purchase your essential oils from, you must do the same research on who is giving you guidance on the safe use of your essential oils. The National Association for Holistic Aromatherapy (NAHA) is one of the leading organizations for establishing guidelines for levels of education for aromatherapy practitioners. There are many countries that do recognize and license aromatherapists. The United States is not one of them. NAHA is a fabulous resource for information on essential oils and their general safe use and is also a good resource for finding schools to take additional training through. NAHA should be the standard to which you hold your aromatherapist when you are seeking guidance. The level I course for certification is a minimum of two hundred hours of instruction, completion of a ten-page research paper, and twenty-five to thirty individual case studies where the student works with clients and the issues they have, develops a blend based on therapeutic properties of essential oils, monitors results, makes modifications, and reports their findings to his or her instructor for feedback. This is just to get a level one certification. There are several advanced levels of training available, but this is the minimum you should be looking for in your aromatherapist.

You are now armed with the information you need to make educated choices when seeking a company to purchase your essential oils from and a practitioner for guidance in the best and safest use to support your body in maintaining balance.

Let's quickly look at four simple rules to follow:

1. *Never* purchase essential oils from eBay or Amazon. You have absolutely no guarantee of what is in that bottle. Replacement caps can be purchased for any size bottle, allowing for someone to refill the bottle with whatever they want and turn around and sell it.
2. Always ask for the GC/MS testing sheets. Even if you don't know what you are looking at, the fact that they are willing to give them to you speaks volumes. Be sure the essential oils were tested in an independent lab, not in-house by the company you are purchasing them from.
3. Find out what type and how much training the person has who is giving you guidance on the safe use of your essential oils.
4. Enjoy. Have fun. Always put safety first.

Safe Use of Essential Oils

Health Risks of Essential Oils

Like anything, too much of a good thing can be bad. There are risks associated with the overexposure of essential oils, but the proper use of them is medically enhancing to our lives. It is always best to use the oils under the guidance of an aromatherapy practitioner. It is also prudent to seek medical attention should you experience any signs or symptoms of overexposure.

Most essential oils were not meant to be ingested. While the oils do have supporting medicinal benefits, they are also highly concentrated. Keep in mind that there are exceptions to this rule of thumb, and knowing what you are putting into your body is critical. For example, chamomile can be used in a tea to ease an upset stomach. It's also important to note that whatever flows into your body gets processed in the liver and kidneys. Too much exposure to chemicals (even the natural ones) can be harmful to organ function.

Many essential oils travel into the body by inhalation. The oil vaporizes into the air in the form of an aroma. You inhale those aromas, and they then enter into your bloodstream to affect our brain and nervous system. Prolonged effects may change the chemical makeup of our tissues. Chemicals are still chemicals no matter whether you can see them or not. What are the side effects of this inhalation? You may feel dizzy or light-headed. You may even experience headaches or nausea. If you have experienced any symptoms like these, step outside to get some fresh air and let your body readjust. Remove the essential oil element and discard it.

Everyone's body reacts differently to different things. If you're also taking medication, using essential oils could impact that treatment.

Essential oils that are topically applied (meaning applied directly to your skin) may also create rash-like symptoms or redness. These symptoms are temporary effects, but exposure to a large enough area could be very irritating to deal with. Safely test to see if your skin can handle the oil application by applying a drop of oil mixed with a tablespoon of vegetable oil to your skin. If the skin turns red or if there is burning or itching, cease the use of the oil immediately and flush the area with a carrier oil to help absorb the essential oil. Consult with your doctor and aromatherapy practitioner. Essential oils that are applied topically can support healing of many skin conditions like acne, eczema, and athlete's foot.

It is especially important that if you have a medical condition or are pregnant or nursing, that you consult with a medical professional before using essential oils. In addition, it is recommended that you read all the safety information before using them.

While there are risks involved, the use of essential oils to promote health and wellness has been a growing market as people seek to find natural methods for treating illness in their body. We find that risks vary from person to person and that moderation is best practice. Remember to be under the guidance of a doctor and/or aromatherapy practitioner while using the oils. Make the most of what nature provides and minimize risk by understanding what is involved and how to correctly use the product.

Robert Tisserand, in my opinion, is the father of safety when it comes to essential use. He has decades of experience and research on this topic. Many of my references will come from his book *Essential Oil Safety*. I take a very safe and conservative approach to my teachings when it comes to using essential oils. You will hear many conflicting reports when it comes to the safe use of essential oils. The ultimate decision is yours on how you will use them. It is my mission to give you the best and most proven methods of incorporating essential oils into your life, so that you can make an educated decision for your health.

Dilution

This is probably the single most controversial topic out there when it comes to essential oils. You may have seen reference material where you are guided to use essential oils undiluted (neat). There may be occasional times where you might want to use an essential oil directly on your skin, without diluting it. I want to stress that this is an exception and not the rule to safe use. I will not cover this method of essential oil use in this book as it should only be done under the guidance of an experienced aromatherapist. Over time, you can build up a tolerance to the chemical components of the essential oil and may no longer see the therapeutic benefits that you once experienced. Skin sensitivity is another major reason I recommend only occasional (when necessary) use of undiluted essential oils. You can develop an adverse reaction when oils are placed directly on your skin. The goal is to achieve the maximum therapeutic benefit with minimal adverse effects.

You will see recommended dilution rates from 0.1 percent to 10 percent. There are no hard and fast rules on dilution rates. One must take into consideration the age and health status of an individual before deciding on a dilution for use. You can never go wrong when you start out with a low concentration and work your way up if you are not seeing the desired results. When diluting, you should always look to a skin-nourishing carrier oil. A carrier oil is the base solution that you will blend the essential oil with before applying it to the skin. There are many different types of carrier oils, and I will go over them in a future chapter.

Determining how many drops to use for which dilution percentage can be a tad bit cumbersome, so I have created an easy reference chart for you. Dilution calculation starts with a one-ounce bottle of essential oil, which contains between five hundred to six hundred drops. The number of drops depends on the consistency of the oil. Some oils are more viscous, and therefore the drops are larger. To make a 1 percent dilution blend, you would use 1 percent of the total drops of oil in the bottle (five to six drops of essential oil). In a one-ounce PET plastic or glass bottle, you would add the five to six drops of essential oil and then fill to the neck with a carrier oil. This gives you one ounce of a 1 percent diluted blend. Once you practice these calculations a few times, they will become easier to do. It never hurts to double check the chart before blending as a best practice. Once you have this one-ounce basic dilution rate down, you can apply this to higher dilution rates and to larger volume blends. For example, if you want to make a 3 percent blend in a five-ounce bottle, you would start with the basic one-ounce calculation for a 3 percent blend, which would be fifteen to eighteen drops and then multiply that by the five-ounce bottle, giving you a total of seventy-five to ninety drops to be placed into the five-ounce bottle to give you a 3 percent diluted blend.

Carrier	1% Dilution	2% Dilution	3% Dilution
1 ounce (30ml)	5-6 drops	10-12 drops	15-18 drops
2 ounces (60ml)	10-12 drops	20-24 drops	30-36 drops
3 ounces (90ml)	15-18 drops	30-36 drops	45-54 drops

These concentrations are based on the assumption that there are five hundred to six hundred drops of essential oil in the average thirty-milliliter (one-ounce) bottle. Dilutions in this chart are not research based and are given solely as a guideline rather than an absolute rule. The heath conditions of the client and the specific particulate of the essential oil are also important factors to be considered when diluting a blend. It is always recommended to consult with a certified aromatherapist before blending.

1% dilutions are recommended for children under 12, seniors and anyone with health challenges, pregnant women and people with compromised immune systems. This is also a very good place to start if you or someone you are blending for has sensitivities to fragrances.

2% dilutions are wonderful for making blends that you will want to use on a regular basis

3% and higher dilutions should be used specifically for acute issues sand are not necessarily recommended for long term use.

<u>Ingestion</u>

This is one of my black-and-white rules in essential oils. There are occasions when ingestion is the best recommended route for the use of essential oils. Before you attempt to use anything internally, I strongly recommend that you consult with and take the advice of a licensed health care professional who specializes in this area. It is not as simple as mixing a few drops of this and a few drops of that into a gel cap and ingesting it. I am sure you would not dream of mixing a few prescriptions medications that have been known to help an issue that you are currently dealing with. The same should hold true with essential oils. I cannot stress enough that you should consult with a naturopathic doctor (ND) or some other licensed naturopathic health care provider in your area before you make the step to take essential oils internally.

<u>Pregnancy</u>

Essential oils are no different than prescription drugs and over-the-counter medications when it comes to their use during pregnancy. Anything that is put into or onto the mom's body during pregnancy will typically cross over to the unborn child through the shared blood supply in the umbilical cord. It is for this very reason that I recommended consulting with a licensed health care professional who is versed in both obstetrics and naturopathic modalities before venturing down the road of using essential oils during your pregnancy. There are many factors that must be taken into account before safely recommending blends and the use of essential oils for the mom and her unborn baby.

Those who have used essential oils before becoming pregnant will probably want to use them during their pregnancy. Some people will want to try them for the first time while expecting. However, it's important to know how to use essential oils safely during pregnancy.

There are many essential oils and blends of oils that just aren't safe to use during pregnancy. Some herbs that are used in cooking should be avoided in their essential oils forms during all nine months of pregnancy. These include basil, bay leaves, sage, thyme, and oregano. Others are clove, marjoram, and wintergreen. Some of the essential oils are safe for use after the first trimester. There are remedies for many of the discomforts of pregnancy. For example, women often have morning sickness that lasts beyond the first trimester. If so, they can breathe in oil of peppermint, spearmint, or lemon.

It is easy to end up feeling tense and full of muscle pain when you are pregnant. If this happens, a massage could be just the thing you need. With the essential oils of lavender and chamomile mixed with jojoba oil, your partner can help ease away that tension.

Commonly, women suffer from swollen ankles and feet during pregnancy. If lavender, cypress, and juniper oils are mixed with jojoba oil, they can used for massage oil. This blend of essential oils can cause the swelling to decrease.

Pregnant women also have muscle cramps in their legs at times. For this, massage oil can be made from the essential oils of lavender and chamomile, just as for any muscle pain. However, with this pain and any pain of the feet and legs, it is important to be careful when doing the massage. Activating pressure points in these areas can possibly induce labor.

Carrying around all that extra weight can make a woman feel quite fatigued. She may have given up coffee and caffeinated soft drinks for the health of her baby. To energize herself, she can mix essential oils of lavender, grapefruit, and orange with jojoba oil. This can be inhaled or rubbed on the solar plexus. Skin eruptions are common during pregnancies. They are uncomfortable and distressing to many women. Several different conditions can be helped by putting a mixture of essential oils and jojoba oil on the affected areas.

The essential oils you should use for dry skin are geranium, lavender, and rose. For inflamed skin, use chamomile. For itchy skin, use a combination of chamomile and lavender. These remedies should soothe the skin and make it smoother. There's just no getting around stretch marks. If you are getting them, though, you might like to have a way to soothe them and keep them from itching. Just put lavender, geranium, and rosewood essential oils in your jojoba oil for massaging.

Do your homework if you are pregnant and want to use essential oils to relieve some of the discomforts associated with pregnancy. After the first trimester, there are certain essential oils that are safe to use. If you are in doubt, consult an expert. It's important to take the safety of you and your baby into account.

According to Tisserand and Young (charts on pp. 152–53, 156), there are approximately fifty essential oils that are contraindicated during pregnancy and another fifteen that should be restricted during pregnancy and lactation. Oils to be avoided include anise, anise (star), araucaria, artemisia vestige, atractylis, birch (sweet), black seed, buchu, calamint, carrot seed, cassie, chaste tree, cinnamon bark, costus, cypress (blue), dill seed, fennel (bitter), fennel (sweet), feverfew, genipi, hibawood, ho leaf (ct. camphor), hyssop, lanyana, lavender (Spanish), mugwort, myrrh, myrtle, oregano, parsley leaf, parsleseed, pennyroyal, rue, sage (dalmatian), sage, (spanish), savin, tansy, western red cedar, wintergreen, wormwood, yarrow (green), and zedoary. Oils recommended to be restricted during pregnancy and lactation are basil (lemon), boswellia papyrifera, campaca (orange) absolute, lemon balm, lemon leag, lemongrass, may chang, melissa, myrtle (honey), merytle (lemon), nastirtium absolute, tea tree (lemon-scented), thyme (lemon), and verbena (lemon).

There are a few essential oils that don't come with a significant amount of precautions. Lavender, frankincense, Roman chamomile, and sweet orange are a few of these oils. Please note that although these oils are considered safe during pregnancy, they should only be used at a 1 percent dilution.

Premies, Newborns, and Children

There is no dispute that, as parents and caregivers of children, you want to protect those precious little lives and do what is best for them. There is a lot of research and vetting done before choosing a medical professional to deliver and care for little ones. Even more research goes into deciding if you will give a prescribed medication or vaccination to your child. So, why is this same amount of research not being done before using essential oils on them? Great question. The answer seems to be guided by the fact that essential oils are natural products and therefore are deemed safe for use on this particular population. One thing is true about that statement. Essential oils that are 100 percent pure essential oils are natural products—with strong and volatile chemical compositions. Everything that is natural, or from nature, is not necessarily good for you.

You may have read that one drop of peppermint essential oil is the same as drinking twenty-six to twenty-eight cups of peppermint tea. With that in mind, who lets their children drink that much peppermint tea in one sitting? Cocaine, marijuana, aspirin, and many other lethal drugs have come from naturally occurring plants, yet we would not dream of giving them to premies, newborns, or children because of the known adverse effects that they have. Don't get me wrong—I am not saying that essential oils are harmful or should not be used. I am saying that they should be used with great caution for all populations. There are several reasons for this statement, and I will explore them for you.

Let's start with the most fragile of this population—our premature babies. Premature babies come into this world as underdogs with many challenges to overcome. We should not add to these challenges by introducing essential oils into their lives during the delicate developmental months that they missed out on in-utero. Many have underdeveloped respiratory, cardiovascular and immune systems. Essential oils are lipid based and therefore metabolized by the liver and excreted by the kidneys. Essential oils and hydrosols should not be used on premature babies.

Full-term newborn babies still have some considerations when it comes to using essential oils. The skin of a newborn does not fully mature until the age of three months. This causes great concern if you are considering a topical application of essential oils as their skin will be much more permeable to the oils and will absorb much more quickly. As mentioned earlier in this book, my approach to the use of essential oils is a very conservative approach and much more conservative when it comes to children. There are many conflicting recommendations on when it is safe to use diluted essential oils with children. I have chosen to take a very safe approach with children under five and only recommend that you use hydrosols, carrier oils, and butters with them.

A child's immune system develops as he or she grows. It is important that you allow the adaptive side to develop naturally. If children are exposed to different bacteria, their immune systems can then recognize these specific antigens and produce antibodies that will protect them from future attacks from that particular pathogen. If essential oils that are high in antibacterial therapeutic properties are regularly used with small children, it could potentially inhibit the body's natural ability to produce much-needed antibodies to protect from future exposures to bacteria. Many parents do not think through to this cellular level simply because they have not been educated about the development of the human immune system. The best combination or exposure of bacteria to support the developing immune system is not fully known. There has been extensive research done on the effects of shortening the infectious period with the use of antibiotics. This research has shown that shortening the cycle and removing the pathogens too soon can ultimately result in decreasing the immune system's memory of that pathogen. If the immune system has no memory of the pathogen, it will not produce antibodies to fight it off if that particular pathogen is introduced into the body at a later time in the child's life. This cycle can ultimately cause a child to be sick frequently with bacteria that the body has not been able to develop antibodies to fight off naturally. I am not saying that there isn't a time and place for both antibiotics and essential oils in a child's life, but I am saying that there should be much thought put into using both of these methods for treating bacterial issues that arise throughout your child's development. Exposing small children to prophylactic use of essential oils that are high in antibacterial properties may not be in the best interest of their developing immune system.

During the steam distillation process, both hydrosols and essential oils are produced. The essential oils float on top of the water in the collective container during the process. Once the oils are removed, the only thing left is the precious hydrosol. Hydrosols have a variety of therapeutic effects, just like essential oils do, but they are at a much lower concentration. Not all hydrosols and essential oils from the same plant part have the same properties. It is for this reason that you will need to research hydrosols specifically for their best use on children. Hydrosols also tend to have much different aromas than their essential oil counterparts. Many carrier oils and butters have very gentle and soothing properties, and I have included many newborn and child safe recipes. When you are using a diffuser in your child's room, it is important to reduce the amount of drops and never leave it running for more than thirty minutes at a time. Another lovely option for newborns and small children is to rub a blend on a caregiver's shoulder and hold the child in that arm and allow them to passively inhale the blend, making sure that the child's skin does not come into direct contact with the blend.

For children five to twelve, it is a bit more safe to use essential oils, but at very low concentrations. I recommend using only a 1 percent dilution for children in this age group when you are looking at a topical use. When blending for children under the age of twelve, you must approach with extreme caution. The overall health of the child is also a very important factor to consider when blending. Several essential oils are contraindicated with many health conditions, and it is always recommended that you consult with a certified aromatherapist before blending for anyone with associated medical conditions. For all intents and purposes, essential oils should be treated in the same manner that prescription drugs are treated. The overall health of the child, any current medications he or she may be on, and the current issue the child is having must all be considered before blending anything for him or her. This same practice also holds true for adults and is the most overlooked component by most people using essential oils.

Phototoxicity

There are several essential oils that can be extremely dangerous if used on skin that will be exposed to direct UV light (this can be direct sunlight or UV from a tanning bed). Typically phototoxic essential oils are going to be from the citrus family and will be cold pressed. Citrus essential oils that are steam distilled do not fall into the category of being at risk for phototoxicity. There are, however, safe blending dilutions for these phototoxic essential oils (Tisserand and Young, p. 86). Bergamot (0.4 percent), lemon (2 percent), lime (.07 percent), grapefruit (4 percent), bitter orange (1.25 percent), mandarin leaf (0.17 percent), cumin (0.4 percent), angelica root (0.8 percent), laurel leaf absolute (2 percent), rue (0.15 percent), and taget (0.01 percent). Any use above these dilution levels will result in a phototoxic blend, and there should be no direct sun exposure for twelve to eighteen hours after application. If you are blending any of the above oils together in a blend to be put on the skin, there are additional precautions. An example of this would be blending lemon and laurel leaf. They both have a maximum dilution of 2 percent. This does not mean that you can use 2 percent dilution of each. You would need to use 1 percent of each to reach a maximum of 2 percent dilution for the blend. If precautions are not taken and safe blending practices are not adhered to, you can expect anything from severe skin irritation to blistering and severe chemical burning of the skin. Extreme caution must be taken when using phototoxic essential oils. Reminder—this applies only to citrus oils that have been cold pressed and does not apply to steam-distilled oils. This also does not apply to blends that are made for wash-off products, such as hand soap, body wash, or shampoos, and it does not apply to essential oils used in a diffuser.

Shelf Life

All essential oils and carrier oils have a shelf life (expiration date). Shelf life varies for each essential oil and for each carrier oil and is not required to be put on the bottle due to this being an unregulated industry. The shelf life time span is determined from the date of distillation for essential oils and production for carrier oils. For this very reason, I will only purchase essential oils and carrier oils from a company that provides complete testing information done by a third party and that has a very good quality control system in place to track different lots that are being sold of the same oil.

I recommend that when you purchase a new essential oil or carrier oil, you use a log book for tracking the oil, date purchased, and expiration date. This will help you keep track of when your oils will be expiring.

Several things will influence the shelf life of a blend you are making. When you blend several essential oils into a carrier oil, the new blend will take on the shortest shelf life of its ingredients. If you are using a water-based ingredient as a carrier, such as a hydrosol or Castile soap, and you are not using a preservative, you should not make more than you will safely use in a two-week period. With no preservative added, your blend will quickly start to grow bacteria. If you are using aloe vera gel, it typically comes with a preservative already in it, but you will need to use caution if you are blending with another water-based carrier for your blend. The choice to use a preservative is completely an individual one. I personally have chosen not to use any preservatives in anything I make. I prefer to keep them natural.

What do you do with expired essential oils? Great question. You can use these essential oils in cleaning blends. They are still great for this use. I just would not recommend putting them in blends to be used on your skin of in your diffuser.

Pet Safety

There is no doubt that pet owners want what is best for their pets. They search on the Internet, read blogs, and read books giving advice on the best remedies for their beloved pets. It is vitally important to know the source of the information you are reading and what you are potentially going to be applying to your pet. Not all that is on the Internet is factual and in the best interest of your pets. Aromatherapy for animals is a very specialized field and should only be trusted to a certified aromatherapist or holistic veterinarian who is well educated in this area.

Essential oils can be used very successfully with canines, equines, and many other animals under the guidance of the right provider. Felines have a challenge that is not seen with other animals. They have very sensitive metabolic systems, and they lack a very important liver enzyme that humans possess that helps them metabolize essential oils. If you are using a diffuser in your home, you can rest assured that you can safely use it with some general guidelines to follow. Always make sure that your pet can safely leave the room that your diffuser is operating in. Never leave a pet locked in a room with an active diffuser. Be sure to keep your home well ventilated, and do not use your diffuser for prolonged periods of time. Essential oils were never meant to be used as room fresheners for hours on end.

If you want to learn more about how you can incorporate essential oils into the healing of issues with your pet, I recommend that you search out a holistic veterinarian who specializes in the use of essential oils. There are many of them out there. Do your research, ask for credentials and references, and make your final choice like you were choosing a pediatrician for your child.

Blending Synergy

When you blend essential oils together, you are looking for a synergistic effect. It would make sense that if three essential oils that are high in antibacterial properties are blended together, you would have a very strong and potent antibacterial blend. On the surface, this seems as if it should be correct. Truth be told, it is not always the case. Some essential oils, when blended with similar property essential oils, can, in fact, have an antagonistic affect. This means that separately the oils may have certain properties, but when mixed together, the chemical composition changes, as will the therapeutic properties of the new blend. This is not always the case, but it is something that needs to be carefully considered when blending oils together. Synergism of blending is a topic that requires much research and is beyond what the intent of this book is. If you are looking to deepen your understanding of blending, I would suggest you read Jennifer Rhind's book *Aromatherapeutic Blending*. This book is a very good reference guide for blending, and I highly recommend it.

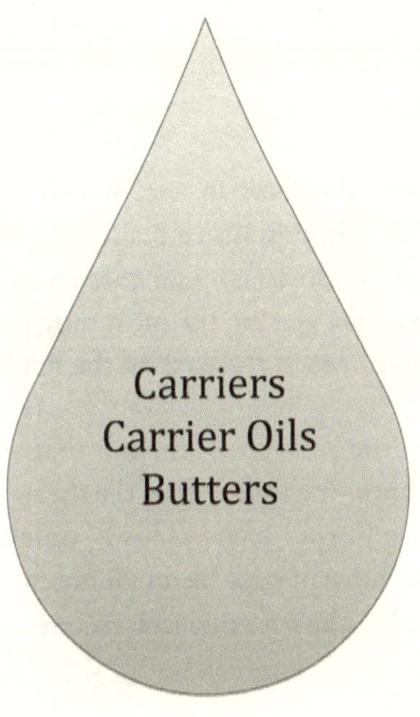

Carriers
Carrier Oils
Butters

As you learned in previous chapters, it is best practice to dilute essential oils before applying them to the skin. Topical application is a wonderful way to not only introduce the essential oils into our body but also an amazing way to help nourish our skin, depending on the carrier we use for dilution. Some of these products can be used on your skin without adding any essential oils as they are hugely beneficial standing on their own merits.

There are dozens of great carriers, carrier oils, and butters that can be used when blending your products. I will share twelve of my personal favorites with you. They all come from various plants, with the exception of beeswax. The fatty acids that are contained in many of them make them fantastic bases for making body products to assist in nourishing and protecting your skin.

When choosing which products to use, it will come down to mostly personal preference. It is important to make sure that you take the same care in choosing where to purchase your carriers, carrier oils, and butters from to ensure that you are getting the most pure products. I have listed a few recommended resources in the back of the book for your use.

Blending will change the shelf life of the oils that you are using. Just as a gentle reminder, your new shelf life will be the shortest shelf life of all of the products you are using in your blend. This is, unless, you are choosing to put an preservative additive in your blend. Some carrier oils are best suited to be kept refrigerated, so be sure to check recommendations for storage.

Aloe Vera Gel

Aloe vera gel is cold pressed from the leaf of the aloe vera plant and has a beautiful translucent white color. This gel permeates the skin barrier very quickly and makes for rapid absorption of blends. Its skin-nourishing and healing properties make it the perfect carrier for hand cleansers, bath products, and facial astringents. On its own, aloe vera gel is an amazing go-to product for burns, as its soothing gel will bring near-instant relief to the burned area. It should not be used on open burns that are associated with second- and third-degree burns.

<u>Argon Oil</u>

Argon oil comes from the nuts of the argon trees of Morocco. It has a slightly golden color and a nutty aroma. The process of preparing the nuts for oil extraction is typically done by hand, and it is very labor intensive. Because of its beautiful golden color and rarity, it is often referred to as "liquid gold." The aroma of this oil is dependent upon when it is harvested. Spring and summer harvests contain a lesser aroma, while fall and winter harvests will have a much deeper nutty aroma. Filled with antioxidants and vitamin E, this carrier oil is an amazing skin-nourishing and moisturizing option when blending essential oils. This carrier oil can be used as the base for hair conditioning, aging, and dry skin blends.

<u>Avocado Oil</u>

Avocado oil comes to us from the oil of the fruit. It is cold pressed and can be found unrefined and refined. Unrefined avocado oil still contains the chlorophyll and brings us a brilliant emerald green color. When the oil is refined, the chlorophyll is taken out and it turns a light brown color but still contains all of the skin nourishing properties that avocado oil is known for. As ambient temperatures start to cool, avocado oil can start to solidify but will return to a liquid state when warmed a bit. Rich in vitamins A, D and E, avocado oil makes for an amazing winter carrier oil base for cracked feet and chapped skin.

<u>Baobab Seed Oil</u>

Baobab oil is cold pressed from the fruit of the adansonita trees, predominately in Africa. The adansonita tree is often referred to as the tree of life due to its ability to hold over eleven hundred gallons of much-needed water in many regions. The fruits also contain high levels of magnesium, potassium, calcium, vitamin C, antioxidants, and omega fatty acids. Its deep golden color and earthy aroma make for a very grounding carrier for all of your skin-healing and nourishing needs as well as bringing valuable vitamins and minerals to your body.

Beeswax

Another wonder of Mother Nature, beeswax comes to us from bees. Their honeycombs are taken from the hives, placed in cheesecloth, and boiled in water. As the honey starts to melt, the wax will seep through the cheesecloth and float on top of the water, bringing with it a wonderful sweet aroma and beautiful rich, golden color. Typically beeswax is not used alone as a carrier but is mixed together with other carriers, such as jojoba, shea butter, cocoa butter, or coconut oil, to add a firmness to products being made such as lip balm or body butters. Being rich in vitamin A, beeswax is a staple in products for the skin to help with cell health.

Cocoa Butter

Cocoa butter, with its pale-yellow color and beautiful cocoa aroma, comes to us from the beans of the cocoa tree. The beans are fermented, roasted, and separated from the hulls. Being a very stable fat, coupled with amazing antioxidant properties, cocoa butter has a shelf life of two to five years. The melting point of cocoa butter is just below human body temperature, making it one of the best carriers for body bars and butters. Its creamy consistency enhances any blend that you may want to use for stretch marks, scars, chapped or burned lips or skin, or itchy skin. If you are looking for a softer product than beeswax will produce, cocoa butter is your go-to carrier.

Coconut Oil

Coconut oil is cold-pressed from the meat of the coconut and is most valuable as a skin-nourishing carrier when it is unfractionated. The fractionation process pulls out all of the nourishing properties but still makes a suitable carrier oil for essential oils. High in saturated fats, coconut oil makes an excellent base for moisturizing hair, nails, and lips as well as an amazing base for dry skin blends. The real beauty of coconut oil is that you can cook with it as well as using it as a carrier oil. At most room temperatures it remains a solid but will liquify when temperatures rise and return back to a solid as temperatures drop. Often blended with jojoba and cocoa butter for lip balms and body butters, coconut oil will bring a chocolaty aroma to your products.

Hemp Seed Oil

Hemp seed oil is generally extracted from industrial hemp plants that typically grow in large-acreage fields close together and can reach twenty feet in height. These plants are very tree like in that they have very fibrous stalks. Hemp oil from these plants does not contain any of the psychogenic properties that come from the marijuana plant. The seeds of the *cannabis sativa* plant are cold pressed and either refined or unrefined. Unrefined is the desired choice so that all of the health benefits remain present. The deep green color and nutty aroma of this oil complement the antioxidant and three-to-one ratio of omega-6 to omega-3 fatty acids. Hemp seed oil assists in balancing our bodies' endocannabinoid system and can help with pain relief, rheumatoid arthritis, eczema, and psoriasis. It makes a great oil for maintaining overall general health, and when blended with complementing essential oils, it can be an amazing supportive addition to one's health.

Jojoba Wax

Jojoba wax comes to us from the beans of the *simmondsia chinensis* plant, which is a shrub-like plant that grows in desert-like climates. Although jojoba is a wax, we sometimes hear it referred to as jojoba oil due to its liquid state at room temperature. It does solidify at cold temperatures and then returns back to its liquid state when warmed, similar to coconut oil. Being a liquid wax, jojoba wax never goes rancid.

It easily penetrates the skin, making for a lovely base for any skin-nourishing blends that you are formulating. Coupled with antioxidant properties, vitamins E and B complex, jojoba wax is a great choice for supporting healthy cells. Infusing into jojoba is very easy, and it allows you to have a variety of scented bases—vanilla, lavender, neroli, and lemon are some beautiful aromas, and they can be used alone or in combination with other essential oils.

Jojoba can also be used as a standalone carrier for makeup removal and skin moisturizer. Fun fact—jojoba oil has been known to be used as a nontoxic pesticide.

Shea Butter

Shea butter is cold pressed from the nuts of the karite trees of Africa. Raw shea butter is a beautiful light yellow color, having a creamy solid consistency. Its triglyceride composition makes for the perfect base for any skin-nourishing product you are looking to make. It has antioxidant and vitamin A and E properties help to support the healing of burned and sun-damaged skin as well as helping with dermatitis, psoriasis, and eczema. With a slightly nutty aroma, shea butter is a great addition for moisturizers, lip balm, and body butters.

Tamanu Oil

Cold pressed from the nuts and fruit of the calophyllum inophyllum trees of Madagascar, tamanu oil bodes a beautiful dark blue-green color with a mildly nutty aroma. Tamanu oil is a highly beneficial oil that can assist with promoting new tissue growth. Full of anti-inflammatory properties as well as antibacterial and antifungal qualities, it can be helpful in keeping those pesky germs away when blended with other like essential oils. Many have been known to use tamanu oil for scar and stretch mark reduction.

Trauma Oil

Trauma oil is an herbal-infused carrier oil with St. John's wort, calendula, and arnica infused typically in olive oil. It's the top gun of carrier oils for any pain or injury blend that you want to develop. The anti-inflammatory and pain-relieving properties of this oil are amazing on their own. When blended with oils like lemongrass, marjoram, lavender, black pepper, or ginger, you can be sure that you will have one very potent blend to help reduce pain and discomfort from both acute and chronic ailments. You can purchase this already blended or try your hand at infusing your own.

In a quart jar, place equal parts of St. John's wort, calendula, and arnica. If you are using fresh herbs, let them wilt for about twelve hours and then cut and crush them with a mortar. If you are using dried herbs, there is no need to crush them. Place the herbs in the bottom of a jar and fill it with olive oil. Leave half an inch of empty space at the top to allow for expansion. Cap the jar tightly and allow it to infuse for three to six weeks. Be sure to place the jar in a warm, sunny spot in your home and shake it gently twice a day. When the infusion process is complete, strain the mixture with cheesecloth and place it in glass jars.

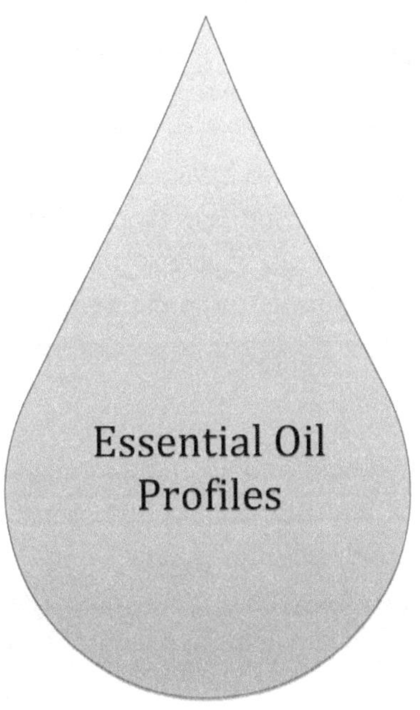
Essential Oil
Profiles

ANGELICA ROOT

Common Name: Angelica root

Latin Name: *Angelica archangelica*

Aroma: Herbaceous, woodsy, earthy

Shelf Life: Four years

Grown by the riverbanks of France, angelica root oil comes to us from the roots of the angelica plant. We can expect this beautiful plant to grow to six feet tall, producing a floral yellow-green blossom in July. Referred to as the oil of angels by many due to its amazing divine healing powers. The Chinese believe it to have may female qualities, helping with menstrual and menopause symptoms as well as being a very strong lymph and blood purifier. When the black plague swept over Europe, the herb was considered an antidote; its seeds and roots were burned to purify the air.

Therapeutic Properties

Angelica and ginger make great companions for digestive issues, specifically gastritis and flatulence. Its analgesic, anti-inflammatory, and antispasmodic properties make it a lovely addition to any injury blend you are making. When you are feeling that annoying chest congestion, consider angelica in a chest rub or inhaler as it can help support healthy lung function.

Emotional Properties

When facing what seems to be an unsurmountable challenge, you can always rely on angelica root to keep you grounded and to strengthen your determination to accomplish the task. Angelica root brings with it balance, calm, and protection to help support a deep and well-rested sleep.

Safety Concerns

Angelica root is phototoxic. According to Robert Tisserand and Rodney Young, the maximum dermal use to avoid phototoxicity is 0.8 percent.

When angelica root is applied at more than this percentage, protect exposed skin from UV rays of sunlight and tanning beds for at least twelve hours. Keep out of the reach of children. If you are pregnant or nursing, consult a physician before use. It should never be used undiluted or internally unless you are under the care of a health care provider trained in the use of essential oils.

Complementary Oils

Blends well with cardamom, sweet orange, balsam fir, and clary sage

BALSAM COPAIBA

Common Name: Balsam copaiba

Latin Name: *Copaifera officianalis*

Aroma: Balsamic, earthy, sweet, warm

Shelf Life: Eight years

This beautiful essential oil comes to us from the amber-colored resin of the balsam copaiba evergreen tree, indigenous to the rainforests of Brazil. These evergreens can grow to over a hundred feet tall and produce a beautiful white flower. A single tree can produce over forty liters of resin annually. The tree does not require harvesting to extract the resin, thereby making this a very sustainable resource for essential oil production. When your muscles are a bit achy, this is one of the go-to oils to help support a reduction in inflammation.

Therapeutic Properties

Balsam copaiba typically contains high percentages sesquiterpenes, which are known for their strong anti-inflammatory properties. In addition to this, it is also anti-analgesic, antibacterial, antifungal, antispasmodic, and antitumoral. This essential oil has been known to support healthy lungs and immune system.

Emotional Properties

Known to quiet the mind and provide a deep sense of tranquilly, copaiba is an incredible oil to use when you need to open and support your root chakra. If you are in need of healing the heart and lifting your mood as well as releasing stuck energy, balsam copaiba is a beautiful addition to your blend.

Safety Concerns

It could cause possible skin sensitivity. Keep out of the reach of children. If you are pregnant or nursing, consult a physician before use. It should never be used undiluted or internally unless you are under the care of a health care provider trained in the use of essential oils.

Complementary Oils

Blends very well with sweet orange, anise, agarwood, frankincense, and cardamom.

BERGAMOT

Common Name: Bergamot

Latin Name: *Citrus bergamia*

Aroma: Lemony, sweet, peppery

Shelf Life: Four years

Bergamot is a very delicate citrus tree grown in southern Italy. The story of how Bergamot landed in Italy is more legend than factual. It is said that Christopher Columbus brought the tree back from the Canary Islands to Spain, and it was from there that it ended up in Calabria, Italy. The trees can grow to ten feet tall at their maturity. Due to damage to the root systems decades ago, trees are now grafted, using buds and branches of bitter orange trees to establish new growth. New growth must mature to at least three years before fruit can be harvested. Typical harvest season is March through May. The rind of the fruit is then cold pressed for extraction of the essential oils. Bergamot is a unique essential oil in that is has both uplifting and calming qualities and makes for a wonderful base for supporting restful sleep.

Therapeutic Properties

Bergamot is known for its antibacterial, antifungal, analgesic, muscle-relaxing, anti-inflammatory, and pain-relieving qualities.

Emotional Properties

It has been known to support deep relaxation, restoration, and calming as well as to support ridding the body of anger and frustration. Bergamot makes a delightful blend for supporting a restful night's sleep and releasing the anxiety of the day.

Safety Concerns

Bergamot must not be applied to the skin undiluted. Serious skin burning or damage can occur if bergamot is applied and the skin is exposed to the sun or a tanning booth. It may be used safely (no phototoxic response) on the skin in a blend at no more than 0.4 percent (approximately one to two drops per one ounce or thirty milliliters of carrier). If oxidized, bergamot essential oil may cause skin irritation or sensitization due to its high limonene content. Keep out of the reach of children. If you are pregnant or nursing, consult a physician before use. It should never be used undiluted or internally unless you are under the care of a health care provider trained in the use of essential oils.

Complementary Oils

Blends well with clary sage, cypress, frankincense, vetiver, and rosemary.

BLACK PEPPER

Common Name: Black pepper

Latin Name: *Piper nigrum*

Aroma: Warm, woodsy, spicy

Shelf Life: Four years

Black pepper essential oil comes from the ripened, dried fruit of the black pepper, commonly found in Africa. The fruit is picked at its maturity, dried, and steamed distilled to bring us an amazing essential oil that has many great benefits. Black pepper has warming qualities that are very welcoming on a cold winter's day when you are headed out for fun and want to give your feet a little extra warm hug with a salve containing this oil. There are some preliminary studies being done looking at the benefits of black pepper in curbing the cravings associated with quitting smoking. Feelings of anxiousness can be reduced as well as supporting a calm digestive system with black pepper.

Therapeutic Properties

It has analgesic, anti-inflammatory, antiseptic, antispasmodic, rubefacient, digestive, expectorant, and vasodilator properties. Black pepper aids in digestion and blends well with ginger and sweet orange for a soothing belly rub after a large meal.

Emotional Properties

It supports mental fatigue and low energy. It can assist in reducing fear that surrounds major life changes. When you are searching for something to help support you with major life decisions or changes, black pepper is a great choice

Safety Concerns

It may be skin irritating. Use it in low dilutions when it is applied to the skin. Do not use it in bath blends. Keep out of the reach of children. If you are pregnant or nursing, consult a physician before use. It should never be used undiluted or internally unless you are under the care of a health care provider trained in the use of essential oils.

Complementary Oils

Blends well with ginger, lemongrass, sweet orange, fennel, frankincense, rosemary, sandalwood, and other spice oils.

BLUE TANSY

Common Name: Blue Tansy

Latin Name: *Tanacetum annuum*

Aroma: Camphoraceous, sweet, and herbaceous

Shelf Life: Four years

This beautiful essential oil comes to us from the yellow-flowered tops of the blue tansy flower, which grows wild in Morocco. The flower tops are steam distilled to bring us an amazing indigo-colored oil that can be of great benefit for supporting the reduction of inflammation and pain management. During insect season, a blend of blue tansy essential oil and Roman chamomile hydrosol makes a delightful spray to help relieve the itch of insect bites. Those suffering with fibromyalgia and arthritis may benefit from this oil. Chamazulene contained in the oil is very skin nourishing. The emotional side of blue tansy can support those who tend to over worry a bit or are stressed easily, as it can help promote relaxation

Therapeutic Properties

It has analgesic, antibacterial, antifungal, antispasmodic, immunostimulant, antiviral, and antioxidant properties.

Emotional Properties

When you are feeling a bit impatient, stressed, or concerned over a situation, blue tansy can help navigate you through to a place of peace and calm. It can be used as a standalone essential oil in an inhaler or blended in a diffuser or body product.

Safety Concerns

Keep out of the reach of children. If you are pregnant or nursing, consult a physician before use. It should never be used undiluted or internally unless you are under the care of a health care provider trained in the use of essential oils.

Complementary Oils

Blends well with helichrysum, German chamomile, and clary sage are complementary oils.

CEDARWOOD

Common Name: Cedarwood

Latin Name: *Juniperus virginiana*

Aroma: Woodsy, earthy, fresh, light

Shelf Life: Eight years

The best analogy for cedarwood is that smell of your grandmother's cedar chest. Feelings of peace, comfort, and calming all come to mind. Cedarwood trees bring us this amazing essential oil through their wood and needles that are steam distilled. This very common tree, found growing wild in the United States, and it is where we get most of our oil from.

Therapeutic Properties

If skin issues are a concern for you, specifically eczema related, you may find great relief from using cedarwood. Conifers in general provide analgesic and anti-inflammatory properties, making them the perfect base for pain and injury blends for those who enjoy the aroma of the outdoors. Although many people with allergies think they should stay away from the conifers because of pollen issues, this is not the case. Cedarwood has very strong lung-supporting properties that can benefit those with deep chest congestion issues. Using a bit of this oil in a water bottle can make for a fabulous insecticide spray.

Emotional Properties

Ever have that project that just won't end and you feel like you cannot go another minute working on it? Well, that is when to pick up cedarwood to help with elevating your mood, giving you that extra boost of confidence, and grounding you to stay the course and finish strong.

<u>Safety Concerns</u>

It is nontoxic. Many sources recommend to avoid during pregnancy. There is no specific research to support this claim with *Cedrus atlantics, Cedrus deodar, or Juniperus virginiana.* The existing uncertainty may be due in part to the many different types of cedarwood trees. Keep out of the reach of children. If you are pregnant or nursing, consult a physician before use. It should never be used undiluted or internally unless you are under the care of a health care provider trained in the use of essential oils.

<u>Complementary Oils</u>

Blends well with bergamot, cinnamon, frankincense, lime and neroli.

CHAMOMILE (GERMAN)

Common Name: German chamomile

Latin Name: *Matricaria recutita*

Aroma: Herbaceous, fruity, strong, sweet

Shelf Life: Five years

Grown in Nepal and England, the German chamomile plant produces a beautiful yellow and white flower used to steam distill the essential oils. Flowers are picked just before they bloom to preserve the precious chemical constituents that bring us amazing therapeutic and emotional properties. The vibrant blue-green colored oil that is produced is in part from the high levels of *azulene* that is contained in it. Producing a rather strong aroma, this essential oil is typically best blended with other oils to achieve an aroma that you will enjoy.

Therapeutic Properties

One of the best-known uses for German chamomile is for its skin-healing properties. Wound management and supporting scar healing are two great benefits of the antibacterial, antifungal, and antiviral qualities of this oil. When combined with aloe vera gel, it makes an amazingly soothing way to help relieve sunburn and minor scrapes and scratches. If you are looking to bring these beautiful qualities to your little ones, under five, you should seek out German chamomile hydrosol as it is much more gentle on their skin and you can spray it directly on, with no dilution.

Emotional Properties

When faced with those situations that surround you with a sense of anxiety or depression, German chamomile can bring back the calming and grounding needed to work through the situation and bring you back to being centered and balanced.

<u>Safety Concerns</u>

It is nontoxic and non-irritating if not oxidized. Oils containing farnesens and alpha-biasabolol (German chamomile) inhibit some metabolizing enzymes (CYP2D6) and could potentiate the actions of some antidepressants such as quididine, fluoxetine, and paraoxetine. Used topically or orally, German chamomile could also have drug interactions with codeine and tamoxifen. Tisserand states that these risks are considered "theoretical" based on the research, meaning, "this safety area is really just beginning to emerge as something to be taken seriously, and Rodney and I have flagged different likely risk areas." Tisserand, Robert and Young, Rodney. *Essential Oil Safety.* 2nd edition, 2014, page 243.

Keep out of the reach of children. If you are pregnant or nursing, consult a physician before use. It should never be used undiluted or internally unless you are under the care of a health care provider trained in the use of essential oils.

<u>Complementary Oils</u>

Blends well withbalsa fir, bergamot, neroli, lemon, frankincense, and lavender.

CHAMOMILE (ROMAN)

Common Name: Roman chamomile

Latin Name: *Chamaemelum nobile*

Aroma: Slightly fruity, sweet, warm

Shelf Life: Five years

Roman chamomile comes to us from the steam-distilled white flowers of this low-growing perennial ground cover. We can see this plant grown in many areas of the world. Its flowers bring an apple or peach-like aroma with them, which makes this oil a great additive to blends. We see these flowers used in teas for bringing a sense of peace and calm. Roman chamomile is much milder than its counterpart, German chamomile, and is a great choice for children and the elderly populations. Its history dates back to ancient Egypt, where it is was known to be a cure for fever. Roman chamomile is one of the most calming and relaxing essential oils available and is very gentle on your skin.

Therapeutic Properties

When you have that tired, sore muscle feeling all over, Roman chamomile can help work through those feelings and bring you back to feeling vibrant and new again. When your tummy is a bit upset or you just finished up with a huge meal, a nice blend with Roman chamomile to rub on your belly may be just the ticket to your digestion challenges. The anti-inflammatory and analgesic properties have traditionally brought supportive pain relief.

Emotional Properties

After a busy and full day, Roman chamomile can help to soothe and calm the worries of the day, and it is great for soaking in a bath before bed to support a restful night's sleep. When you need a little extra dose of patience, you can turn to Roman chamomile to bring peace and harmony back into a situation.

Safety Concerns

Keep out of the reach of children. If you are pregnant or nursing, consult a physician before use. It should never be used undiluted or internally unless you are under the care of a health care provider trained in the use of essential oils.

Complementary Oils

Blends well with bergamot, clary sage, grapefruit, lemon, lavender, and neroli.

CINNAMON BARK

Common Name: Cinnamon bark

Latin Name: *Cinnamomum zeylanicum*

Aroma: Spicy, sweet, warm, exotic

Shelf Life: Five years

Cinnamon bark oil is steam distilled from the bark of the Ceylon tree. This tropical evergreen is indigenous to India, Madagascar, and Sri Lanka and can grow to forty-five feet in height. Being very rich in cinnamaldehyde, it is not like most other essential oils that are rich in aldehydes. Cinnamon bark oil is a "hot" oil, which means it should be used topically with extreme caution and in very low dilution rates. It is recommended to use one drop in forty milliliters of carrier oil when blending for topical use. It should never be used in any bath products or put directly on the skin undiluted. This essential oil is particularly best suited for diffuser use.

Therapeutic Properties

According to the ORAC scale, which is the measurement scale for concentration of antioxidants in foods, cinnamon is ranked number seven. While supporting metabolic function, cinnamon bark is also a good supporter of the immune system and has amazing air-purifying qualities. With its warm and spicy aroma, it makes for a wonderful addition to winter diffuser blends.

Emotional Properties

Cinnamon bark oil brings with it very grounding and uplifting properties, as well as restoring balance and a sense of well-being.

Safety Concerns

This oil should be used very cautiously on the skin. It can cause burning and blistering as well as contact dermatitis. Dilution rates should also be very conservative—one drop per forty milliliters. It should not be used during pregnancy or while nursing or with children under five years of age. Use care when diffusing as it can be irritating to sensitive eyes. Keep out of the reach of children. If you are pregnant or nursing, consult a physician before use. It should never be used undiluted or internally unless you are under the care of a health care provider trained in the use of essential oils.

Complementary Oils

Blends well with bergamot, frankincense, lavender, lemon, orange, and rosemary.

CLOVE BUD

Common Name: Clove bud

Latin Name: Eugenia caryophyllata

Aroma: Fruity, spicy, sweet, warm

Shelf Life: Four years

Clove bud oil comes to us from the steam distillation of delicate, unopened crimson buds of the Eugenia caryophyllata evergreen. This beautiful tree is native to southeast Asia. Its warm, spicy aroma blends amazingly well with sweet orange, ginger, cardamom, and opopanax for a delightful fall/winter potpourri blend. In ancient Greece and Rome it was used to soothe toothaches and to combat unwanted breath odors.

Therapeutic Properties

The dominant chemical constituent in clove bud oil is eugenol, which it has proven anti-inflammatory properties. When we see inflammation reduced, typically pain relief follows. It is for these two properties that this oil makes a great addition to blends that are looking to support pain relief, reducing inflammation. The rubefacient properties help to support increased circulation, which will help to bring fresh oxygenated blood to painful, sore, and inflamed areas.

Emotional Properties

There is great emotional support that can be gained from clove bud oil. The spicy nature of this essential oil brings with it a sense of self-confidence. If it is more energy to tackle a big challenge, you can count of clove bud oil to help you climb that challenging mountain.

Safety Concerns

The eugenol present in clove bud oil is thought to be inhibit monoamine oxidase (MAO), which is found in antidepressant drugs. Great caution should be used for people who are taking MAO inhibitors and selective serotonin reuptake inhibitors (SSRI) medications. Topical use dilutions should be limited to 0.5 percent, and clove bud oil should be avoided in children. Keep out of the reach of children. If you are pregnant or nursing, consult a physician before use. It should never be used undiluted or used internally unless you are under the care of a health care provider trained in the use of essential oils.

Complementary Oils

Blends well with bergamot, cardamom, ginger, opopanax, and sweet orange.

CORN MINT

Common Name: Corn mint

Latin Name: *Mentha arvensis*

Aroma: Fresh, minty, herbaceous

Shelf Life: Five years

Corn mint, also known as wild mint, grows in the temperate regions of Europe, Asia, Himalaya, Siberia, and North America. The leaves of this plant are steam distilled to bring us an essential oil that has many of the same properties as peppermint essential oil. When kept at cooler temperatures, corn mint oil has a tendency to crystalize, but with a quick dip of the bottle into a container of warm water, it will return to its liquid state.

Therapeutic Properties

When you want to manage minor pain, inflammation, and muscle spasms, corn mint oil can help support with its analgesic antispasmodic properties. The carminative properties in corn mint are known to help support symptoms associated with irritable bowel syndrome and to promote overall digestive health.

Emotional Properties

For days when you just cannot seem to shake the blues, reach for corn mint. Its uplifting and mood-balancing properties can help you to promote a positive outlook and turn that frown upside down. When it is time to put a little pep in your step for a big test or meeting, mix a little corn mint with rosemary and lemon to help you bring your A game.

Safety Considerations

According to Tisserand and Young, corn mint oil should be avoided in people with atrial fibrillation and G6PD deficiency. It should also be avoided in anyone who is currently taking anticoagulants due to menthol being a known anticoagulant. It is not to be used with anyone on calcium channel blockers. It should be avoided in children under five and with anyone suffering with gallbladder issues. Keep out of the reach of children. If you are pregnant or nursing, consult a physician before use. It should never be used undiluted or internally unless you are under the care of a health care provider trained in the use of essential oils.

Complementary Oils

Blends well with bergamot, balsam copaibo, lavender, lemon, rosemary, and sweet orange.

ELEMI

Common Name: Elemi

Latin Name: Canarium luzonicum

Aroma: Citrus, warm, woodsy, spicy, exotic

Shelf Life: Three years

Elemi oil comes to us from the steam-distilled, pale yellow resin of the Pili tree of the Philippines. These trees thrive in extreme heat accompanied by torrential rains. The more the tree is jostled by the wind, the more abundant the fruit crop is. Pili trees are tapped in a self-sustaining manner to extract the resin in a manner that does not harm the tree. Ancient Egyptians found that the antiseptic properties of elemi oil made it an excellent option for embalming.

Therapeutic Properties

Elemi oil provides some of the same benefits as frankincense and myrrh and is an amazing skin-nourishing product. When you are looking for an essential oil for an anti-aging skin blend, this is a must ingredient. It can help support tone and firm the skin while reducing wrinkles and fine lines. Elemi oil, when added to a bath blend, can help to sooth those overtaxed muscles from a hard workout.

Emotional Properties

Combined with frankincense, elemi oil makes for an amazing meditation blend. It brings a sense of grounding and balance to the room and will help with clearing your root chakra of stuck energy.

<u>Safety Concerns</u>

Keep out of the reach of children. If you are pregnant or nursing, consult a physician before use. It should never be used undiluted or internally unless you are under the care of a health care provider trained in the use of essential oils.

<u>Complementary Oils</u>

Blends well with black spruce, grapefruit, frankincense, myrrh, and neroli.

EUCALYPTUS GLOBULUS

Common Name: Eucalyptus globulus

Latin Name: *Eucalyptus globulus*

Aroma: Camphoraceus, fresh, sweet, earthy, woodsy

Shelf Life: Four years

Eucalyptus globulus essential oil comes from the steam-distilled leaves of the eucalyptus tree, which is native to Madagascar, Spain, Portugal, Brazil, and Chile. Ancient Aborigines were said to have used eucalyptus leaves to wrap wounds, treat body pains, relieve sinus congestion, fever, and colds. Most eucalyptus globulus is made up of between 80 to 90 percent 1.8 cineole, which is a powerful oxide. In the 1880s surgeons used it for its antiseptic properties.

Therapeutic Properties

Due to its extreme high content of 1.8 cineole, we tend to see airborne antimicrobial, analgesic, antibacterial, antioxidant, antispasmodic, antiviral, dopaminergic, increased cerebral blood flow, and mucolytic property benefits with this essential oil. At the first sign of a cold, you can use a steam to help support your body in ridding itself of the germs. Eucalyptus globulus is used in many spa and personal care products. It is a great supporter of our respiratory system and can help with those pesky muscle and joint aches.

Emotional Properties

Having properties that support cerebral blood flow and mental clarity, this essential oil blends great with rosemary and lime for those times when you want to be on top of your game. Being able to clear out negative thinking and bring back an uplifting sense of peace is another amazing benefit of eucalyptus globulus

<u>Safety Concerns</u>

If it is oxidized, it can cause irritation. It should not be used with babies or children under ten years old on their face or inhaled with steam or personal inhaler. Great care should be taken with asthmatics. Keep out of the reach of children. If you are pregnant or nursing, consult a physician before use. It should never be used undiluted or internally unless you are under the care of a health care provider trained in the use of essential oils.

<u>Complementary Oils</u>

Blends well with frankincense, lavender, and rosemary.

FENNEL

Common Name: Fennel

Latin Name: *Foeniculum vulgare*

Aroma: Sweet, fresh, earthy, anisic, spicy

Shelf Life: Four years

Indigenous to the Mediterranean shores, the fennel plant's seeds are steam distilled to bring us an essential oil that is soothing to the mind and body. Believed to grant strength and courage to ancient Egyptians and Romans, garlands of fennel were worn to give praise for their victories. When we think of fennel, we think of the strong and present aroma of anise, which brings with it strong digestive support.

Therapeutic Properties

The predominant anethole properties that fennel have provide analgesic, anti-inflammatory, anticoagulant, antifungal, antithrombotic, antiulcerogenic, antiviral, and sedative support. Fennel's most well-known supportive property is for digestion. It can help relieve constipation, nausea, and bloating. Support of the lymphatic system is recognized from the anti-inflammatory characteristics.

Emotional Properties

When you are feeling a bit creatively stuck, fennel can support getting your creative juices flowing again. Supporting our ability for clear and confident communications is another beautiful quality of fennel.

Safety Concerns

It is advised for short term use and at maximum dilution strengths of 2.5 percent. It should not be used in children under five years of age. It is contraindicated in pregnancy and breastfeeding. It is not advised to be used during labor. Keep out of the reach of children. If you are pregnant or nursing, consult a physician before use. It should never be used undiluted or internally unless you are under the care of a health care provider trained in the use of essential oils.

Complementary Oils

Blends well with geranium, ginger, grapefruit, lemon, sweet basil, and sweet orange.

FRANKINCENSE

Common Name: Frankincense

Latin Name: *Boswellia carterii*

Aroma: Pine, woody, lemon, spicy

Shelf Life: Three years

Frankincense has a history that dates back some five thousand years and has many biblical references. The boswellia sacra tree grows in Somalia, Arabia, Ethiopia, and Sudan and is known to grow in some of the most rugged environments. Once a tree reaches the age of eight to ten years, it can be tapped by slashing the bark and allowing the precious resin to bleed out. As the resin is released and dries, it makes a teardrop-looking substance. The trees can be tapped multiple times throughout a year. The more opaque the resin, the better the quality. It is important to read the gas chromatography results for frankincense since it can be either rich in monoterpene oils or ester oils.

Therapeutic Properties

Not many essential oils have better skin-healing properties than does frankincense. Scars respond very nicely to topical application. Due to the chemical constituents of pinene, d-limonene, and myrcene, we find great analgesic benefits as well as anti-inflammatory and antioxidant properties. Frankincense is always a good go to oil when you are stuck trying to decide what to blend.

Emotional Properties

Strong grounding qualities come as a result of the amazing ability the boswellia sacra tree has to wrap its roots around rocks and grow up through them. Frankincense is known for its ability to support mind clearing, increase concentration, and ease impatience. Many yoga studios use frankincense for its deep meditation properties.

Safety Concerns

Keep out of the reach of children. If you are pregnant or nursing, consult a physician before use. It should never be used undiluted or internally unless you are under the care of a health care provider trained in the use of essential oils.

Complementary Oils

Blends well with clove, lavender, lemon, lime, myrrh, sweet orange, tea tree, and vitiver.

GINGER

Common Name: Ginger

Latin Name: *Zingiber officinale*

Aroma: Warm, spicy, lemony, woody, balsamic

Shelf Life: Five years

Rhizomes, or roots, of the beautiful ginger plant bring us a lovely and aromatic essential oil. Madagascar, Thailand, China, and India are all homes to the ginger plant. Using a steam distillation process to bring out the oils, ginger is most well-known for its support of a healthy digestive system. While we most commonly see ginger used in Asian cooking, Native American cultures have been known to use ginger essential oils to help regulate menstruation and heartbeat. When you are using it as a topical application, always consider blending with a skin-nourishing essential oil to help balance the potential skin irritation qualities of ginger.

Therapeutic Properties

Ginger has been used in Western medical practice for many years to aid relief of digestive issues as well as for its pain-relieving qualities. Nausea is one of the many digestive challenges that ginger assists with as well as providing support of an overall healthy digestive system. Pain and inflammation can also benefit from the use of ginger.

Emotional Properties

The warmth of ginger brings out so many wonderful emotionally supporting qualities. Feeling a little like you are burning the candle at both ends and something has to give? That's the time to reach for ginger essential oil. Blend it with something uplifting from the citrus family to bring your motivation back to a place of "I can conquer the world."

<u>Safety Concerns</u>

Keep out of the reach of children. If you are pregnant or nursing, consult a physician before use. It should never be used undiluted or internally unless you are under the care of a health care provider trained in the use of essential oils.

<u>Complementary Oils</u>

Blends well with cinnamon, grapefruit, lemon, sweet orange, frankincense, and bergamot.

HELICHRYSUM

Common Name: Helichrysum

Latin Name: *Helichrysum italicum*

Aroma: Fruity, sweet, herbaceous, rich

Shelf Life: Five years

Coming to us from the rocky mountains of the Mediterranean, *helichrysum italicum* is in the daisy family. It is often referred to as a curry plant due to the strong aroma its leaves give off. It is not to be confused with the spice curry used in cooking, as they are not one in the same. These beautiful plants, with their golden yellow flowers can grow upwards of twenty-four inches. The amazing wound-healing properties of this essential oil come from the steam distillation of the plant's flowers. This may be, by far, the best essential oil to use for wound management and skin healing. Helichrysum has had many studies done on its antimicrobial and wound-healing properties.

<u>Therapeutic Properties</u>

If you have little ones, this is an essential for the essential oil first-aid kit. From the pesky bug bite to scraps and scratches that children get, helichrysum can help support the healing process. The reaction to just one undiluted drop on a wound is amazing. It is almost instantaneously that we start to see healing. Lavender and frankincense are wonderful follow-up essential oils to help support the continued healing process. Spasms associated with cough, overworked muscles, and irritable bowel syndrome can all benefit from a blend made with helichrysum.

<u>Emotional Properties</u>

The wound healing doesn't stop with surface injuries. For all of those old emotional wounds that are buried deep inside and causing you unrest, reach for helichrysum to bring balance and harmony back to your spiritual world.

<u>Safety Concerns</u>

Do not use on puncture wounds. Wait until the skin has healed back together before use. Keep out of the reach of children. If you are pregnant or nursing, consult a physician before use. It should never be used undiluted or internally unless you are under the care of a health care provider trained in the use of essential oils.

<u>Complementary Oils</u>

Blends well with lavender, clary sage, rose, citrus, and spice oils.

HEMLOCK

Common Name: Hemlock

Latin Name: *Tsuga candenis*

Aroma: Piney, woodsy, coniferous, balsamic, warm

Shelf Life: Three to four years

Tsuga candenis is a mighty conifer that can grow to heights of seventy feet and a span of thirty-five feet. It is native to North American and Canada and not to be confused with the toxic hemlock, which comes from a completely different species and genus. Cool, damp ecosystems close to water are where these amazing trees grow. Most grow to the ripe old age of four to five hundred years, with the oldest living hemlock at one thousand years old. Like most of our conifers, the hemlock gives us wonderful respiratory support accompanied with immune and adrenal support.

Therapeutic Properties

Hemlock loves to support a healthy respiratory system with its mucolytic, expectorant, and decongestant properties. Caution should be used with anyone who has asthma or chronic respiratory issues and slowly introduce this essential oil by taking a gentle sniff from the bottle to see how you react. If any respiratory discomfort or chest tightness is experienced, this would not be a good choice for you. Hemlock blends well in a chest rub, inhaler, or diffuser.

Emotional Properties

When your chakras are feeling a bit unbalanced, hemlock can help clear many of them for you. Hemlock can bring the energy back to your sacral chakra, unconditional love into your heart chakra, ability to speak your truth to your throat chakra, and heightened perception back to your third eye chakra. Rest with hemlock to relax and bring order back to a chaotic and stressful day.

<u>Safety Concerns</u>

Use caution with anyone who has asthma or chronic respiratory issues (as noted above). Keep out of the reach of children. If you are pregnant or nursing, consult a physician before use. It should never be used undiluted or internally unless you are under the care of a health care provider trained in the use of essential oils.

<u>Complementary Oil</u>

Blends well with rosemary, lavender, clary sage, and cedarwood.

JUNIPER BERRY

Common Name: Juniper berry

Latin Name: *Juniperus communis*

Aroma: Piney, fresh, resinous, earthy, sweet

Shelf Life: Three years

Native to Europe, Asia, and parts of North America, the *juniperus communis* produces a blue/violet berry-like cone that is harvested in early Autumn and steam distilled to bring us juniper berry essential oil. In early Greek and Arabic times, juniper tea was used by physicians to disinfect their surgical instruments. Western European cultures would plant the juniper berry bush by their front doors to keep witches from entering. Tibetans used juniper to remove demons. In today's culture, we most commonly see juniper berry used to make gin. Gin gets its name from the Dutch word *jenever* and the French word *genievre*, which both translate to the word *juniper*.

Therapeutic Properties

Juniper berry essential oil supports many areas of our body. Assisting to support increased circulation and reducing fluid retention, juniper berry works to reduce pain and inflammation and makes a wonderful addition to massage blends. When you are looking for an essential oil to use to support healthy lung function, this oil works great in a chest rub.

Emotional Properties

When you are headed down the rabbit hole of worry and overwhelm, reach for juniper berry to help you restore calm and peace to those situations. If clearing your mind and spirit are what you need for the day, it can also assist with that process.

Safety Concerns

Keep out of the reach of children. If you are pregnant or nursing, consult a physician before use. It should never be used undiluted or internally unless you are under the care of a health care provider trained in the use of essential oils. Be mindful of the species of juniper berry you are using, as some can be contraindicated during pregnancy and with kidney disease.

Complementary Oils

Blends well with bergamot, cypress, grapefruit, lavender, lemon lime, rosemary, and sweet orange.

LAVENDER

Common Name: Lavender

Latin Name: *Lavendula angustifolia*

Aroma: Herbal, woody, fresh, balsamic

Shelf Life: Six years

Lavender is one of the most common of the essential oils and one that is used by many for its immediate calming properties. We see lavender used in many bath and body products as well as food products. Lavender is grown in India, South France, Italy, Bulgaria, and many places in North America. The beautiful blue/violet flowers of the lavender plant are steam distilled to bring us what many refer to as their go-to essential oil. Lavender can be beneficial in most any situation and blends well with so many other essential oils. Just walking through a lush lavender field brings a soothing sense of peace and tranquility.

Therapeutic Properties

The main chemical constituent in lavender is linalol, which has been studied extensively and has much scientific data to support its many benefits to supporting our health and wellness. Linalol is most well-known for its analgesic, anti-inflammatory, antibacterial, antioxidant, and immunostimulant properties. Lavender hydrosol can be used directly on the skin of adults and small children. It makes a great "boo-boo" spray for those cuts and scrapes. Spray a bit of lavender hydrosol on a baby's crib sheet or blanket about twenty minutes before napping or retiring for the evening to bring a sense of peace and calmness.

Emotional Properties

Linalol combined with linalyl acetate have been known to sedate the central nervous system, which is what makes lavender such a sought-after essential oil for supporting a restful night's sleep. Lavender brings an overall sense of wellbeing, balance, love, and peace with it.

Safety Concerns

Keep out of the reach of children. If you are pregnant or nursing, consult a physician before use. It should never be used undiluted or internally unless you are under the care of a health care provider trained in the use of essential oils.

Complementary Oils

Blends well with bergamot, clary sage, frankincense, sweet orange, and tea tree.

LEMON

Common Name: Lemon

Latin Name: Citrus limon

Aroma: Fresh, clean, citrus, cheery

Shelf Life: Two years

Lemon essential oil comes to us from cold pressing the rind of the fruit of the lemon trees. Much of our supply of lemon essential is imported from Italy. We are all familiar with the general use of lemons in our everyday life. We make lemonade, pies, breads, and cakes and even cook with lemons. Lemon, as an all-natural household cleaning product, is a fabulous use for lemon essential oil.

Therapeutic Properties

Lemon essential oil is d-limonene, which is known to activate white blood cells. Analgesic, anti-inflammatory, antibacterial, anti-obesity, antioxidant, antitumoral, immunostimulant, and anti-anxiety are all properties of d-limonene, which makes lemon essential an amazing oil to add to blends. Its cooling properties bring a lovely support to pain relief and inflammation.

Emotional Properties

The fresh aroma that lemon essential oil brings with it sets the stage for bringing joy, happiness, and positive energy. Used in a room diffuser or a personal inhaler, you can always count on lemon essential oil to lift that funky cloud from over you and bring you back to a positive and uplifting state of mind.

<u>Safety Concerns</u>

Cold-pressed lemon essential oil is phototoxic and should always be used in low concentrations if you are using it topically and are planning on going out into the sun or using a tanning bed within eighteen hours of application. If you use a dilution of less than twelve drops per ounce (30 ml), you will not have those same phototoxic effects. If using in a topical or bath blend with no worry of UV exposure, you should use no more than a 1—2 percent dilution due to possible skin irritation. Keep out of the reach of children. If you are pregnant or nursing, consult a physician before use. It should never be used undiluted or internally unless you are under the care of a health care provider trained in the use of essential oils.

<u>Complementary Oils</u>

Blends well with eucalyptus, fennel, frankincense, peppermint, sandalwood, and sweet orange.

LEMONGRASS

Common Name: Lemongrass

Latin Name: *Cymbopogon citratus*

Aroma: Lemony, herbal, grassy, earthy

Shelf Life: Four years

Lemongrass is a perennial plant native to India, Guatemala, and Indonesia, which can grow to heights of three feet. Light, sandy soil with moist and warm climates are where you will find this bright green, grassy plant. Lemongrass essential oil comes from the steam distillation of partially dried leaves, which are roughly textured with sharp edges. Yellow/amber in color, this essential oil has many wonderful therapeutic properties. Lemongrass itself is popular in many culinary delights of Thailand, Vietnam, and Indonesia.

Therapeutic Properties

Citral being a main component of lemongrass essential oil contributes to its antifungal effects. Anti-inflammatory and analgesic properties make this essential oil a staple for many massage therapy practices to help with muscle soreness. The antipyretic properties help with supporting fever reduction.

Emotional Properties

Lemongrass can be very soothing and mind calming for those times when you just need to put the cares of the day behind you. For those times when you seem "stuck" in a place of not moving forward, lemongrass can help move you through this period in time.

Safety Concerns

Can cause irritation to skin and mucous membranes. Maximum dilution should not exceed 0.7 percent. During pregnancy, Tisserand recommends not using over a 0.5 percent dilution so not to affect fetal development. Essential oils high in citral should be avoided with antidepressants. Keep out of the reach of children. If you are pregnant or nursing, consult a physician before use. It should never be used undiluted or internally unless you are under the care of a health care provider trained in the use of essential oils.

Complementary Oils

Blends well with basil, black pepper, cedarwood, juniper, lavender, palmrosa, sandalwood, and vetiver.

MANDARIN

Common Name: Mandarin

Latin Name: *Citrus reticulata*

Aroma: Fruity, sweet, fresh, citrusy

Shelf Life: Three years

Mandarin essential oil comes to us from cold pressing the rind of the fruit. There are two varieties of mandarin, and although they are comparative in therapeutic properties, they differ in aroma. Mandarin (green) comes from the very young fruit that is not ripe and has a more tart, crisp aroma. Mandarin (red) comes from the fully ripened fruit and presents with a more sweet aroma. Mandarin essential oil has been used in traditional Chinese medicine since AD 400. Historically, it was a traditional gift given to Imperial Chinese officials.

Therapeutic Properties

Mandarin essential oil has an abundance of wonderful properties. It is best known for its ability to help support a healthy digestive system, specifically to help with nausea. Included in its multifaceted properties are antioxidant and antiseptic as well as assisting to reduce scars and stretch marks.

Emotional Properties

During meditation, if you feel your chakras are filled with blocked energy, mandarin diffused during this time can help to release this blocked energy. Supporting courage and bringing an uplifting tone to your mood are both qualities that this essential oil brings to the table.

Safety Concerns

Keep to a maximum of 1 percent dilution for topical use. Keep out of the reach of children. If you are pregnant or nursing, consult a physician before use. It should never be used undiluted or internally unless you are under the care of a health care provider trained in the use of essential oils.

Complementary Oils

Blends well with lavender, ginger, and sweet marjoram.

MARJORAM (SWEET)

Common Name: Marjoram (sweet)

Latin Name: *Origanum marjorana*

Aroma: Pine, spicy, citrus, warm, woodsy

Shelf Life: Four years

Sweet marjoram essential oil comes to us from the beautifully aromatic green flowers and leaves of the perennial marjoram herb that are steam distilled. Indigenous to France, Spain, and South Africa, marjoram is a symbol of joy and happiness in many ancient cultures. The Greek and Romans used it for decorating both weddings and funerals.

Therapeutic Properties

Antibacterial, antiseptic, analgesic, antispasmodic, anti-inflammatory, digestive-stimulating, and immune supporting are some of the many properties of this essential oil. It is especially helpful for reducing muscle spasms and calming the central nervous system. Blended with peppermint and sweet orange for a sports massage lotion is a favorite of many massage therapists for treating those overworked muscles.

Emotional Properties

For those times when you need to let the guard down around your heart, yet you don't quite feel safe enough to do just that, marjoram can help calm and protect you. When dealing with emotional grief, it can help bring comfort to mind and spirit.

Safety Concerns

Keep out of the reach of children. If you are pregnant or nursing, consult a physician before use. It should never be used undiluted or internally unless you are under the care of a health care provider trained in the use of essential oils.

Complementary Oils

Blends well with blue tansy, black pepper, bergamot, lemongrass, sweet orange, and peppermint.

MELISSA

Common Name: Melissa

Latin Name: *Melissa officinalis*

Aroma: Lemony, citrus, fresh, floral

Shelf Life: Four years

The bright green, mint-like leaved melissa plant is common to Europe and South Africa. A frost-hardy plant, it prefers full sunlight unless the temperatures are unseasonably hot. Then it prefers partial sun. This very rare and precious essential oil requires over sixty pounds of plant material to make just one five-milliliter bottle of oil. The flowers and leaves are steam distilled to make a beautiful essential oil that is used for supporting many areas of our life.

Therapeutic Properties

Melissa essential oil brings many rejuvenating properties. In ancient times, this oil was used for calming nervous disorders and to promote fertility. Antidepressive, antiviral, sedative, antispasmodic, and antibacterial are some of the supportive therapeutic properties melissa offers. The sedative qualities of melissa are second to none and should be used cautiously. Its anti-inflammatory and analgesic qualities make for a wonderful addition to pain relief blends. Insomniacs can benefit from a more restful night's sleep when using melissa.

Emotional Properties

Often referred to as the elixir of the heart, melissa does well in helping to pacify anger and give comfort during extremely stressful times. Balance and uplifting are two qualities that are dominant and help to bring peace and calmness.

<u>Safety Concerns</u>

Avoid using with children under two years of age. May interfere with diabetes medication if taken internally. Use should be restricted to 0.5 percent topically during pregnancy due to the possible effects of citral in fetal development, according to Tisserand.

<u>Complementary Oils</u>

Blends well with geranium, lavender, palmrosa, and vetiver.

NEROLI

Common Name: Neroli

Latin Name: *Citrus aurantium var. amara*

Aroma: Citrus, floral, sweet

Shelf Life: Four years

Neroli dates back to seventeenth-century Italy when Ann Marie Orsini, duchess of Bracciano and princess of Nerola, used essence of bitter orange in her baths and on her gloves. Since that time, it has been referred to as neroli. The largest producers of neroli essential oil are Morocco and Tunisia, where the delicate blossoms are hand-picked in late April to early May. The bitter orange tree brings us three beautiful essential oils. Neroli from the blossoms, petitgrain from the leaves and twigs, and bitter orange from the rind. Neroli is one of our very precious and rare essential oils. Over one hundred pounds of blossoms are used to make just one pound of essential oil. Take care when choosing a supplier for this oil, as it is one that is frequently adulterated.

Therapeutic Properties

Neroli typically has high concentrations of d-limonene and linalol. From the linalol, we see analgesic, anti-inflammatory, and antibacterial properties that make this a wonderful addition to blends for pain, inflammation, and muscle spasms. D-limonene also supports these same ailments, along with antibacterial properties.

Emotional Properties

D-limonene's anti-anxiety properties make this the perfect oil for helping to support situation depression, emotional struggles associated with loss, and heartache. Using a drop mixed with a small amount of carrier oil and rubbed in the heart chakra area will help clear stuck energy.

Safety Concerns

Keep out of the reach of children. If you are pregnant or nursing, consult a physician before use. It should never be used undiluted or internally unless you are under the care of a health care provider trained in the use of essential oils.

Complementary Oils

Blends well with bergamot, frankincense, lemon, myrrh, palmrosa, sandalwood, and sweet orange.

OPOPANAX

Common Name: Opopanax

Latin Name: *Commiphora guidotti*

Aroma: Warm, woodsy, rich, vanilla-like, floral

Shelf Life: Four years

Opopanax essential oil is a close cousin to myrrh essential oil and is often referred to as sweet myrrh. They share therapeutic properties but their aroma differs greatly. Growing in the dry climates of Somalia, the resin of the *commiphora guidottiixi* tree is steam distilled into a yellowish-red oil. Opopanax has been traditionally used in Somalia and Eritrea. They have played a role in women's initiation rites—to help heal the physical scars of female circumcision and to cleanse, disinfect, and tighten the womb after birth. It is common for this essential oil to separate in the bottle, causing small crystals to form. Both the oil and the resin can be used for incense.

Therapeutic Properties

Having high amounts of monoterpenes and sesquiterpenes, opopanax brings with it decongesting, anti-inflammatory, and antispasmodic qualities. It has been known to balance digestion and lessen lung congestion due to its drying qualities. Cicatrisant properties give opopanax beneficial skin-healing properties, and we see it used frequently in skin care products.

Emotional Properties

Meditation rituals are a very common place for the use of opopanax. The grounding and deep relaxation qualities make for a beautiful incense blend to be used during yoga or meditation. Unblocking stuck energy is one of the many ways that this oil brings harmony and balance.

<u>Safety Concerns</u>

According to Tisserand and Young, opopanax can have skin-irritating qualities and should be used at low dilution concentrations (1 percent). Keep out of the reach of children. If you are pregnant or nursing, consult a physician before use. It should never be used undiluted or internally unless you are under the care of a health care provider trained in the use of essential oils.

<u>Complementary Oils</u>

Blends well with grapefruit, juniper, lavender, spikenard, and sweet orange.

ORANGE (SWEET)

Common Name: Orange (sweet)

Latin Name: *Citrus sinensis*

Aroma: Fruity, fresh, citrus

Shelf Life: Two years

Sweet orange essential oil comes to us from the cold-pressed rind of ripened sweet oranges. South Africa, Italy, and China are countries that bring us much of the world's supply of sweet orange. Nothing says "pick me up" better than the sweet, citrus aroma of orange. Its d-limonene properties bring with it wonderful antibacterial properties, making it a wonderful base for natural cleaning products.

Therapeutic Properties

Extremely high in d-limonene, sweet orange presents with analgesic, anti-inflammatory, antibacterial, antioxidant, anti-tumoral, anti-ulcerogenic, immunostimulant, and anti-anxiety properties. Mixed with lavender and peppermint, you can have a beautiful blend for easing minor pain and inflammation for sore muscles. If it is used in an inhaler, you can bring relief to an upset tummy after a big meal or relief from nausea.

Emotional Properties

The uplifting, cheery, and bright aroma that sweet orange has will help turn your frown upside down. When the room needs a bit of peace and joy, you can always count of this oil to support bringing a sense of positivity and relaxation.

Safety Concerns

Sweet orange is not phototoxic but should be used in lower-dilution concentrations (1 to 2 percent). Citrus products are typically heavily sprayed with pesticides, so be sure to find an organic source for your oils. Keep out of the reach of children. If you are pregnant or nursing, consult a physician before use. It should never be used undiluted or internally unless you are under the care of a health care provider trained in the use of essential oils.

Complementary Oils

Blends well with cinnamon bark, frankincense, lavender, lemon, peppermint, and sandalwood.

PALO SANTO

Common Name: Palo santo

Latin Name: *Bursera graveolens*

Aroma: Balsamic, rich, sweet

Shelf Life: Three years

The mystical palo santo tree is grown in Ecuador and Peru and has a very unique harvesting process. The precious essential oils do not produce in these trees until at least two years after they naturally die and have fallen. Trees cannot be harvested live for their oils. After sufficient time has lapsed from the time of the tree's death, the oil is steam distilled from the wood of the tree. Often referred to as "holy wood," indigenous people of the Amazon have used it in cleansing and healing rituals, similar to sage and cedar. It has been said to bring good fortune to those who are open to its magic. The smoke of the burning wood is very helpful at keeping mosquitos and other insects away.

Therapeutic Properties

D-limonene properties of this oil bring amazing anti-infectious qualities that help support the body in times of colds, flu, and infection. The skin-nourishing qualities of palo santo make it a top choice for blending skin-care products.

Emotional Properties

Hundreds of years after the shamans burned palo santo in their rituals and ceremonies, many have continued to use this amazing space clearing essential oil in their homes to promote the flow of positive energy. Enhancing creativity, focus, and concentration make this a wonderful choice for those times when you are feeling a little blocked and scattered.

Safety Concerns

Keep out of the reach of children. If you are pregnant or nursing, consult a physician before use. It should never be used undiluted or internally unless you are under the care of a health care provider trained in the use of essential oils.

Complementary Oils

Blends well with frankincense, myrrh, and sandalwood.

PEPPERMINT

Common Name: Peppermint

Latin Name: *Mentha x piperita*

Aroma: Mentholic, fresh, strong, herbaceous, minty

Shelf Life: Five years

Peppermint is one of the more common essential oils, which has a very strong aromatic presence. It brings true meaning to the phrase "a little dab will do you." Just opening the bottle and taking a gentle sniff can sometimes be enough to ward off the beginning stages of a headache or nausea or the need for a pick-me-up. Steam distilled from the leaves of the peppermint plant, this essential oil is best known for its digestive qualities but has many attributes that it brings to the table. It dates back to the Egyptian pyramids of 1000 BC. Peppermint, mixed with orange or lemon in a small bottle of distilled water, makes for an amazing kitchen or bath cleaning spray.

Therapeutic Properties

High in menthol and menthone properties, we see high degrees of analgesic, anti-inflammatory, antibacterial, antispasmodic, cooking, and Central Nervous System (CNS) stimulating qualities in peppermint. Overworked or stressed muscles can benefit from a blend made of peppermint, lavender, and orange. Peppermint in a personal inhaler is always good to have with you when you feel a headache coming on. If you have been on your feet all day, a lovely foot bath with Epsom salt, Himalayan sea salt, jojoba oil, and a little peppermint essential oil will be just what your tootsies need.

Emotional Properties

There is nothing better than peppermint essential oil to give you that midafternoon energy boost that you need to get you through the rest of the day. It has been known to sharpen your mind and keep you focused on the task at hand when blended with rosemary and lime.

Safety Concerns

May cause skin and mucous membrane irritation, and it is recommended that 2 percent of less dilution concentrations be used when making topical blends. Keep out of the reach of children. If you are pregnant or nursing, consult a physician before use. It should never be used undiluted or internally unless you are under the care of a health care provider trained in the use of essential oils.

Complementary Oils

Blends well with grapefruit, lavender, lemon, lime, rosemary, and sweet orange.

RAVINTSARA

Common Name: Ravintsara

Latin Name: *Cinnamomum camphora ct 1.8 cineole*

Aroma: Fresh, clean, eucalyptus-like

Shelf Life: Four years

Cinnamomum camphora is an evergreen tree, commonly found in Madagascar to heights of sixty to ninety feet. It produces a glossy, waxy leaf that smells of camphor when crushed. In the spring, these trees produce a beautiful white flower with clusters of black, berry-like fruit. Ravintsara essential oil comes to us from the steam distillation of the leaves and typically has very high concentrations of 1.8 cineole, which can cause central nervous system and breathing issues in young children. Like lavender, ravintsara *is a very* universal essential oil.

Therapeutic Properties

Essential oils that are high in 1.8 cineole bring with them qualities that include: antimicrobial, anti-inflammatory, antibacterial, antioxidant, antispasmodic, mucolytic, antiviral, and immune supporting. These qualities make ravintsara a wonderful oil for muscle aches and pains as well as giving great support for headache relief. It is a go-to oil when making winter blends to help combat cold and flu symptoms. Many who suffer with shingles find great relief from itching and pain.

Emotional Properties

When in need of focus and clarity in times of stress and tension, ravintsara can help by supporting an increase in cerebral blood flow. It is also known to help calm a nervous and anxious mind.

<u>Safety Concerns</u>

Tisserand and Young remind us that essential oils that are high in 1.8 cineole can cause central nervous system (CNS) and breathing problems in children and are not recommended for children under ten years of age. Keep out of the reach of children. If you are pregnant or nursing, consult a physician before use. It should never be used undiluted or internally unless you are under the care of a health care provider trained in the use of essential oils.

<u>Complementary Oils</u>

Blends well with cedarwood, cinnamon bark, eucalyptus, lavender, lemon, peppermint, and rosemary.

SANDALWOOD

Common Name: Sandalwood

Latin Name: *Santalum album*

Aroma: Woodsy, musky, sweet, earthy

Shelf Life: Eight years

Sandalwood trees grow abundantly in Hawaii, India, Indonesia, and Australia. Caution must be given to the potential of over harvesting these precious trees for their oils. Sandalwood essential oil comes from steam distilling the wood of the tree. Trees must be a minimum of fifteen years old to be used for this purpose. The older the tree, the more and better quality the oil is. Being the second-most-expensive wood in the world, it is in high demand. With this in mind, one must be careful where one is purchasing sandalwood essential oil, as it can often be adulterated.

Therapeutic Properties

Due to the high levels of both alpha and beta sanatol, sandalwood gives great support to promoting healthy skin and hair and can be used in skincare and haircare products. It also brings us anti-inflammatory properties that can help support reducing minor pain and muscle spasms.

Emotional Properties

Sandalwood brings with it great emotional grounding and protection qualities, making it a wonderful essential oil for times when deep meditation is desired. When self-acceptance and balance are needed, reach for sandalwood.

Safety Concerns

This oil is very commonly adulterated. Be sure that you can access the gas chromography testing results before you purchase sandalwood. Keep out of the reach of children. If you are pregnant or nursing, consult a physician before use. It should never be used undiluted or internally unless you are under the care of a health care provider trained in the use of essential oils.

Complementary Oils

Blends well with frankincense, lemon, myrrh, spruce, and ylang.

SITKA SPRUCE

Common Name: Sitka Spruce

Latin Name: *Picea sitchensis*

Aroma: Pine, woodsy, earthy, balsamic, resinous

Shelf Life: Four years

Sitka spruce trees can be found in southeast Asia, Canada, Oregon, and Iceland, just to name a few, but there are only a few distillers who produce essential oils, and they are mostly in France. These magnificent trees can reach heights of over 330 feet, with their trunks growing to over 16 feet in diameter. It is the largest spruce tree in the world and the fifth-largest conifer in the world. They can grow to be the ripe old age of five hundred–plus years and love wet climates. Sitka spruce essential oil comes to us from the steam distillation of the needles.

Therapeutic Properties

Sitka spruce is extremely high in a-myrcene and b-myrcene, which are both known for their analgesic and anti-inflammatory properties. These properties make this oil a great candidate for blends to help support reducing pain, inflammation, and muscle tension. It also brings with it antiviral, antibacterial, and antimicrobial properties for helping to support your body during cold and flu season to reduce mucus, aches, and pains. It you love the smell of walking through the woods, you can make an amazing cleaning product with this oil.

Emotional Properties

If you are looking to restore and revitalize after a stressful situation or a taxing week at work, a diffuser blend that includes sitka spruce will do the trick. When you are looking to boost your self-confidence and self-image, you can count on this essential oil to help.

Safety Concerns

Keep out of the reach of children. If you are pregnant or nursing, consult a physician before use. It should never be used undiluted or internally unless you are under the care of a health care provider trained in the use of essential oils.

Complementary Oils

Blends well with bergamot, cypress, grapefruit, juniper, palo santo, ravintsara, and vetiver.

SPIKE LAVENDER

Common Name: Spike lavender

Latin Name: *Lavandula latifolia*

Aroma: Camphoraceous

Shelf Life: Five years

Lavandula latifolia often gets confused with *lavandula angustifolia*. The two are very different in chemical properties. *Lavandula angustifolia* is best suited for its calming affects, whereas *lavendula latifolia* is better suited for times of bringing a more energetic mood. *Lavandula latifolia* is high in both linalol and 1.8 cineole. Spike lavender has similar qualities to eucalyptus, peppermint, and ravintsara.

Therapeutic Properties

Spike lavender has significantly more camphor than does lavender, and it is also high in linalol and 1.8 cineole, which make it a great addition to blends for supporting pain relief and reducing inflammation. Headaches respond very well to spike lavender. Its mucolytic, antibacterial, antiviral, and airborne antimicrobial properties allow for support of respiratory issues such as congestion and spastic cough.

Emotional Properties

Helping to promote alertness and reduce fatigue are one of the benefits you can achieve from this essential oil. It also can help to calm anxiety and stress with its uplifting qualities.

Safety Concerns

Tisserand and Young suggest using spike lavender with caution for anyone suffering from epilepsy. Although the camphor content is not high enough to be contraindicated during pregnancy, it is best advised to avoid spike lavender during pregnancy. Keep out of the reach of children. If you are pregnant or nursing, consult a physician before use. It should never be used undiluted or internally unless you are under the care of a health care provider trained in the use of essential oils.

Complementary Oils

Blends well with eucalyptus, frankincense, peppermint, and rosemary.

TULSI

Common Name: Tulsi

Latin Name: *Ocimum sanctum ct eugenol*

Aroma: Earthy, fresh, minty, spicy, warm

Shelf Life: Four years

Tulsi or holy basil, as it is frequently referred to, comes to us from the steam distilled flowers and leaves of a very specific variety of the basil plant of India. In India, Ayurvedic medicine refers to it as the "elixir of life." The woody stalks are commonly used for making meditation and rosary beads. Tulsi is known as an adaptogen, which enables the body to be brought into balance with its use.

Therapeutic Properties

Tulsi is rich in beta caryophyllene, a cannabinoid that specifically works on the

CB2 pathways in our body and brings with it support for helping with inflammation, pain, atherosclerosis, and osteoporosis through our endocannabinoid system in our body. Phenols are known for their ability to stimulate the immune system and are highly anti-infectious.

Emotional Properties

As an adaptogen, tulsi is greatly beneficial in bringing your mood back to balance. Its warm and uplifting properties help to bring a sense of self-confidence and self-assurance.

Safety Concerns

High eugenol and phenol properties bring with them caution when used in topical applications. It is recommended that a 1 percent or less dilution concentration is used. It should not be used in bath products and should not be used with babies or children. Tulsi should not be used in an inhaler and should not be used undiluted on the skin. According to Tisserand and Young, oils high in eugenol should be used with caution on those with impaired liver function and not used at all in people who have clotting disorders, as eugenol is an anticoagulant. Keep out of the reach of children. If you are pregnant or nursing, consult a physician before use. It should never be used undiluted or internally unless you are under the care of a health care provider trained in the use of essential oils.

Complementary Oils

Blends well with bergamot, clary sage, geranium, lemon, and lime.

VETIVER

Common Name: Vetiver

Latin Name: *Vetiveria zizanoides*

Aroma: Earthy, balsamic, smoky, sweet

Shelf Life: Eight years

Vetiver essential oil comes to us from the steam-distilled root of this perennial grass that is native to India. Grasses can grow to heights of five feet, and the strength of their immense root system grows straight down to depths of ten feet. This plant is very drought tolerant and helps with soil erosion. Vetiver is a very viscous essential oil and can be hard on diffusers. It is best used topically with a carrier oil. The aroma of this oil is very strong and tends to be a love it or leave it oil. It is always best to take a test smell of this essential oil before purchasing it to make sure it is one that you will enjoy.

Therapeutic Properties

Vetiver has amazing skin-nourishing qualities as well as anti-inflammatory properties. A warm bath is a great place to bring vetiver, diluted with a carrier such a jojoba. It can soothe the minor aches and inflammation of arthritis, rheumatism, sore muscles, and muscle tension. Supporting your immune system is also a quality that vetiver brings. The skin-nourishing abilities make for a wonderful ingredient for topical blends to help with eczema, acne, and wound care.

Emotional Properties

One of the most well-known qualities of vetiver is its ability to help support insomnia, anxiety, and depression. Coming from the root of its plant, it brings with it very strong emotionally grounding affects. When your root chakra is feeling a bit stuck and you need an energy shift, you may want to consider taking a walk out in nature after putting a small dab of a blend vetiver on your wrists or behind your ears to help get that stuck energy flowing again.

Safety Concerns

Keep out of the reach of children. If you are pregnant or nursing, consult a physician before use. It should never be used undiluted or internally unless you are under the care of a health care provider trained in the use of essential oils.

Complementary Oils

Blends well with lavender, lemon, sandalwood and sweet orange

My Favorite Recipes

In this section, I will bring you some of my favorite recipes for using essential oils. As mentioned earlier in the book, I have a very safe approach when it comes to using essential oils with babies and small children. I do not advocate the use of essential oils for anyone under the age of five and only a 1 percent dilution concentration for children five to twelve. This is not a hard and fast rule, just the angelic energy approach for the safety of our children. For anyone under five years of age, I recommend using hydrosols for helping support their bodies. These are very effective and extremely safe for even newborns. When I am considering making blends or using essential oils for anyone who is on medication or chronically ill, I always recommend consulting with their physician or licensed naturopathic healthcare professional before introducing essential oils.

When making your recipes, always be sure to use glass containers for mixing, glass rods for stirring, and glass or PET plastic for storing your recipes. Expiration dates for your blends will be the expiration date of the ingredient that is soonest to expire. It is always recommended to make only what can be used in a few weeks, unless you are planning to add a preservative to your blends. Preservatives are not covered in this book, as it is my intent to keep our recipes all natural.

Inhaler blends are designed for personal use by an individual, not to be shared. There are several options for an inhaler to use. Check that resource section for a list of trusted vendors. When making an inhaler, you will place the cotton wick into the inhaler tube, place essential oil drops onto the cotton wick, and then place the bottom cap into place. Place a label on the tube, and you are all set. Inhalers typically will last for two to three months before you will have to make a new one. PET plastic ones are disposable, and glass insert inhalers are designed for reuse.

When you are making a stock blend of a recipe, you are making a large quantity of the blend so that when you want to make an inhaler, lotion, bath salt, or any other form of application, you will have all the ingredients perfectly blended, and all you will have to do is put the appropriate number of blend drops into your application based on the dilution concentration you want to achieve. These are good to make for blends that you use frequently.

For carrier oil based blends, you can substitute the carrier used in the blend recipe for any carrier oil that you like. Some carrier oils are used because they have specific therapeutic qualities themselves. For example, trauma oil is frequently used in pain blends due to its own ability to help support pain relief all by itself.

For diffuser blends, it is recommended that you refer to the manufacturer's recommendations for amount of drops to use in your reservoir, as there are many different sizes that will require different amounts.

KID-SAFE RECIPES

FOR NEWBORNS TO FIVE YEARS OF AGE

Rock-A-Bye Baby Linen Spray

1 ounce Roman chamomile hydrosol
1 ounce lavender hydrosol

Combine the ingredients in a glass or PET plastic bottle. Spray on bedding ten minutes before putting your little one down to sleep. You can also spray on a caregiver's shoulder while rocking to help promote sleep.

Rub-A-Dub-Dub Bath Oil

1/2 ounce frankincense hydrosol
1/2 ounce lavender hydrosol

Add to bathwater just before placing child into tub. This blend is both skin nourishing and relaxing for your little one.

Baby Bum Diaper Cream

1/4 cup shea butter
1/4 cup coconut oil
1 T beeswax
1 T bentonite clay
2 drops Roman chamomile hydrosol
2 drops lavender hydrosol

In a double boiler or glass bowl, melt beeswax and then add coconut oil and shea butter. Once everything is melted, remove it from heat and add bentonite clay and hydrosols and stir gently with a glass rod. Pour into a small glass or PET plastic container. Allow it to cool for twenty-four hours before using. Use during diaper changes to help soothe away irritation.

Cradle Cap Oil

1 tsp. jojoba wax
2 drops helichrysum hydrosol

Mix the ingredients together in the palm of your hand and gently rub on your baby's scalp.

Tummy Tonic

1 ounce fennel hydrosol
1 ounce Roman chamomile hydrosol

Combine the hydrosols in a glass or PET plastic spray bottle. When your baby is struggling with colic, spray a few sprays on the baby's tummy and rub in a clockwise motion. Be careful not to get spray onto your baby's face

Baby Powder

1 ounce white kaolin, white clay
1 tsp. arrow root
1 tsp. vanilla bean powder
1 tsp. Roman chamomile flowers

Place flowers in a new (never used) coffee grinder or food processor until they are ground into a fine powder. Add to the clay and mix with a glass stirring rod. Place the mixture in a container and use it during diaper changes to soothe the baby's skin.

Skin-Nourishing Baby Oil

1 cup apricot kernel oil
2 T calendula flowers
2 T lavender flowers

Place calendula and lavender flowers in a glass jar and fill with oil. Place the lid on the jar, and keep it in a cool, dry place for six to eight weeks. Shake the jar twice a day during the six to eight weeks. This makes an amazing oil, and it is safe for your baby's skin.

Soothing Baby Lotion

1/2 cup jojoba oil
1/4 cup coconut oil
1/4 cup beeswax
1 T shea butter
1 T cocoa butter

Combine jojoba oil and beeswax in a double boiler. Once these are liquified, add coconut oil, shea butter, and cocoa butter. Stir occasionally during this process. Once it is completely melted, pour it into a glass jar or tin for storage. This blend does not dispense well in a pump or squeeze container. It is wonderful for use with babies, children, and adults, as this is a very skin soothing and nourishing blend. Best if used within two to three months, as it has no preservatives.

Baby Stain Remover

4 ounces distilled water
1 T borax
10 drops lemon essential oil

Mix the ingredients in a glass or PET plastic spray bottle. Gently shake the mixture and then spray directly on the stain and wash.

FOR CHILDREN FIVE TO TWELVE YEARS OF AGE

Relaxing Body Oil

2 ounces jojoba wax
4 drops lavender
6 drops cedarwood
2 drops bergamot

Sore Muscle Support

2 ounces trauma oil
4 drops marjoram
3 drops lavender
3 drops basil

Relaxing Bath Blend

Add no more than 2 drops of essential oil to a tablespoon of carrier oil.

1 drop lavender
1 drop cedarwood

Or

1 drop ylang ylang
1 drop vetiver

Cold Season Personal Inhaler

4 drops sweet orange
3 drops lavender

Place a cotton wick into the inhaler base, drop oil onto the wick, and pop on the base cap. Your child is now ready to use his or her own personal inhaler to help ward off those cold and flu bugs.

Nourishing Skin Lotion

8 ounces unscented lotion
15 drops cedarwood
10 drops sweet orange
10 drops helichrysum
5 drops lavender

Ouch Away

2 ounces of distilled water
4 drops lavender
2 drops cypress
4 drops helichrysum

Fill a glass or PET plastic spray bottle with distilled water, and add the essential oil drops. Place the spray top on and give a little shake. Spray on minor cuts and scrapes.

DIGESTION SUPPORT

Tummy Tamer Lotion

8 drops ginger essential oil
6 drops lavender essential oil
4 drops peppermint essential oil

Add drops to lotion or carrier oil and rub on the tummy in a clockwise motion every few hours.

No More Nausea Inhaler

7 drops peppermint essential oil
4 drops sweet orange essential oil
5 drops mandarin essential oil

Irritable Bowel Syndrome Support

10 drops sweet orange essential oil
6 drops lavender essential oil
8 drops Roman chamomile essential oil
4 drops sandalwood essential oil

Add drops to two ounces of lotion or carrier oil and apply to the abdomen every few hours.

Gas Be Gone

8 drops bergamot essential oil
4 drops ginger essential oil
3 drops cardamom essential oil
5 drops rosemary essential oil

Add drops to two ounces of lotion or carrier oil and apply before or after meals

Heartburn Inhaler

7 drops lemon essential oil
6 drops peppermint essential oil
3 drops sandalwood essential oil

Place a cotton wick into the inhaler chamber, add essential oil drops, and place a cap on the bottom of the inhaler chamber. Use every twenty minutes for supporting relief.

Cranky Constipation

6 drops peppermint essential oil
5 drops ginger essential oil
4 drops tarragon essential oil
6 drops fennel essential oil
8 drops anise essential oil

Add to two ounces of lotion or carrier oil and rub on the abdomen in a clockwise motion every few hours.

STRESS, ANXIETY, AND INSOMNIA SUPPORT

Sleepy Time Roller Ball

5 drops sandalwood essential oil
7 drops lavender essential oil
5 drops German chamomile essential oil
4 drops frankincense essential oil
8 ml jojoba oil

Add drops to a ten-milliliter roller ball container and then add jojoba oil. Place the roller ball cap tightly on the container, gently shake it, and you are ready for use. Rub on your wrists or behind the ears about twenty minutes before retiring for the evening.

Sleep Away Diffuser Blend

1 ml lavender essential oil
2 ml bergamot essential oil
1 ml mandarin essential oil

Place drops of oil in a five-milliliter oriface reducing bottle. Use approximately ten drops in your diffuser. This stock blend can also be used for an inhaler by placing fifteen drops onto the cotton wick of a new inhaler set.

Peaceful Sleep Blend

10 drops vetiver essential oil
6 drops lavender essential oil
4 drops wild orange essential oil
4 drops mandarin essential oil

Add to two ounces of lotion or carrier oil and rub a small amount behind the ears, forehead, and temples before retiring for the night.

Mental Stress Booster Stock Blend

2 ml rosemary essential oil
1 ml lime essential oil
1 ml sweet orange essential oil

This stock blend can be used for making inhalers and topical blends with lotion or carrier oils or can be used in a diffuser. It will help to support mental clarity and reduce mental fatigue.

Stress Be Gone Inhaler

5 drops elemi essential oil
4 drops lavender essential oil
3 drops melissa essential oil
4 drops sweet orange essential oil

Place a cotton wick into the chamber of a new inhaler set, and add drops onto a cotton wick, secure the bottom cap, and you are all set to help combat stress throughout your day with your own personal inhaler to use anytime you need support.

Ditch Your Anxiety

14 drops spike lavender essential oil
8 drops German chamomile essential oil
6 drops rosewood essential oil
4 drops sandalwood essential oil

Add to two ounces of lotion or carrier oil.

Serenity Stock Blend

1 ml lavender essential oil
1 ml marjoram essential oil
1 ml ylang ylang essential oil
1 ml sandalwood essential oil
1 ml neroli essential oil

Place the ingredients in a five-milliliter oriface reducing bottle. The mixture can be used for making a personal inhaler, for topical applications, or in a diffuser.

Ahhhh Roller Ball

7 drops cypress essential oil
5 drops Roman chamomile essential oil
4 drops clary sage essential oil
30 ml jojoba oil

Place the essential oil drops into an empty roller ball container, and add jojoba oil. Securely place the roller ball top on the container, and gently shake it.

Christine Stalsonburg

Get Fired up Stock Blend

1 ml ginger essential oil
2 ml peppermint essential oil
1 ml sweet basil essential oil

Place in a five-milliliter oriface reducing bottle. The mixture can be used for making a personal inhaler, for topical applications, or in a diffuser.

CHAKRA-CLEARING BLENDS

Crown Chakra Stock Blend

2 ml cardamom essential oil
1 ml myrrh essential oil
1 ml rosemary essential oil
1 ml juniper berry essential oil

Place the ingredients in a five-milliliter oriface reducing bottle. The mixture can be used for making a personal inhaler, for topical applications, or in a diffuser. Refer to the dilution chart.

Third-Eye Chakra Stock Blend

3 ml frankincense essential oil
1 ml bergamot essential oil
1/2 ml clary sage essential oil
1/2 ml eucalyptus essential oil

Place the ingredients in a five-milliliter oriface reducing bottle. The mixture can be used for making a personal inhaler, for topical applications, or in a diffuser. Refer to the dilution chart.

Throat Chakra Stock Blend

3 ml sweet orange essential oil
1 ml patchouli essential oil
1 ml German chamomile essential oil

Place the ingredients in a five-milliliter oriface reducing bottle. The mixture can be used for making a personal inhaler, for topical applications, or in a diffuser. Refer to the dilution chart.

Heart Chakra Stock Blend

2 ml neroli essential oil
1 ml palmrosa essential oil
1 ml spikenard essential oil
1 ml geranium essential oil

Place the ingredients in a five-milliliter oriface reducing bottle. The mixture can be used for making a personal inhaler, for topical applications, or in a diffuser. Refer to the dilution chart.

Solar Plexus Chakra Stock Blend

1 1/2 ml laurel leaf essential oil
1 1/2 ml thyme linolol essential oil
1 ml sweet basil essential oil
1 ml clove bud essential oil

Place the ingredients in a five-milliliter oriface reducing bottle. The mixture can be used for making a personal inhaler, for topical applications, or in a diffuser. Refer to the dilution chart.

Sacral Chakra Stock Blend

3 ml ylang ylang essential oil
1 ml lemon essential oil
1 ml peppermint essential oil

Place the ingredients in a five-milliliter oriface reducing bottle. The mixture can be used for making a personal inhaler, for topical applications, or in a diffuser. Refer to the dilution chart.

Root Chakra Stock Blend

2 1/2 ml vetiver essential oil
1 1/2 ml cedarwood essential oil
1 ml opoponax essential oil

Place the ingredients in a five-milliliter oriface reducing bottle. The mixture can be used for making a personal inhaler, for topical applications, or in a diffuser. Refer to the dilution chart.

PAIN RELIEF SUPPORT

Arthritis Support

8 drops helichrysum essential oil
8 drops German chamomile essential oil
8 drops juniper berry essential oil
4 drops ginger essential oil
4 drops lavender essential oil
3 drops mandarin essential oil

Add to two ounces of trauma oil, unscented lotion, or any other carrier of your choice.

Neuropathy Support

10 drops spike lavender essential oil
9 drops black pepper essential oil
6 drops lemongrass essential oil
6 drops clove bud essential oil
4 drops ginger essential oil

Add to two ounces of trauma oil, unscented lotion, or any other carrier of your choice.

Sciatic Support

7 drops spike lavender essential oil
7 drops sandalwood essential oil
6 drops helichrysum essential oil
6 drops frankincense essential oil
4 drops clove bud essential oil
4 drops ginger essential oil

Add to two ounces of trauma oil, unscented lotion, or any other carrier of your choice.

General Pain Support Inhaler

4 drops lavender essential oil
4 drops juniper berry essential oil
4 drops frankincense essential oil
4 drops lemon essential oil

Place a cotton wick into the chamber of a new inhaler set, add drops onto the cotton wick, and secure the bottom cap.

Sore Muscle Tamer

10 drops tulsi essential oil
4 drops spike lavender essential oil
3 drops helichrysum essential oil
3 drops sandalwood essential oil

Add to one ounce of trauma oil, unscented lotion, or any other carrier of your choice.

Sore Throat Support

5 drops myrtle (red) essential oil
5 drops sandalwood essential oil

Add to one ounce of jojoba oil and apply to the exterior throat area.

Acute Pain Relief Support

3 drops cinnamon essential oil
4 drops black pepper essential oil
7 drops lavender essential oil
6 drops elemi essential oil
3 drops sandalwood essential oil

Add to one ounce of trauma oil and apply to affected area. This is a 4 percent blend that is to be used with healthy adults for only a few days. Do not cover the area or apply direct heat to the area after application.

Bug Bite Relief Support

8 drops blue tansy essential oil
5 drops peppermint essential oil
8 drops spike lavender essential oil
3 drops tulsi

Add to one ounce of lavender hydrosol to a PET plastic or glass spray bottle and spray as needed for relief support. Gently shake the bottle before use to ensure a blending of the essential oils and hydrosol.

Headache Support Inhaler

5 drops lavender essential oil
6 drops frankincense essential oil
2 drops rosemary ct. camphor essential oil
1 drop eucalyptus globulus essential oil

Place a cotton wick into the chamber of a new inhaler set, add drops onto cotton the wick, and secure the bottom cap. For adults only.

Muscle Soothing Bath Salt

2 drops frankincense essential oil
2 drops Roman chamomile essential oil
1 drop neroli essential oil
1 tsp. jojoba wax
1 oz. Himalayan sea salt
1 oz. Epsom salt

Fill a two-ounce glass jar with salts, and add essential oil drops and jojoba wax. Stir the mixture with a glass stirring rod until all ingredients are blended. Add the mixture to a water stream in a bathtub just before getting in. Use caution getting out of the tub, as the oils will leave a slippery residue on the bottom of the tub.

Big Guns Pain Support

5 drops copaiba essential oil
5 drops frankincense essential oil
5 drops balsam fir essential oil

Add to one ounce of unscented lotion or carrier oil of your choice, and stir until all oils are blended. Use on the affected area every few hours to support pain relief.

RESPIRATORY SUPPORT

Chest Rub Stock Blend—Daytime

40 drops eucalyptus globulus for adults—radiata for children essential oil
40 drops tea tree essential oil
16 drops thyme linolol essential oil
20 drops ravintsara essential oil

Place the essential oils in a five-milliliter oriface reducer bottle. Use three to six drops of stock blend with a half teaspoon of carrier oil of your choice and massage into chest (front and back) two to three times a day. Use caution not to get the blend near the face.

Chest Rub Stock Blend—Nighttime

40 drops frankincense essential oil
40 drops lavender essential oil
15 drops coriander essential oil
21 drops tea tree essential oil

Place the essential oil in a five-milliliter oriface reducer bottle. Use three to six drops of the stock blend with a half teaspoon of the carrier oil of your choice and massage into the chest (front and back) two to three times a day.

Vanilla Cold Relief Support

12 drops balsam fir essential oil
3 drops sweet orange essential oil

Add to one ounce of vanilla-infused jojoba wax. Apply every couple of hours to help support cold relief.

BATH AND BODY

Solid Stick Deodorant

20 drops lime essential oil
40 drops mandarin essential oil
12 drops lemon essential oil
1 oz. beeswax
2 oz. hemp oil
1 oz. coconut oil

On a stove in a double boiler with glass insert, melt the beeswax, and then add coconut oil and hemp oil. Mix with a glass stirring rod until it is completely melted. Remove from heat, add essential oils, and stir and pour into deodorant containers. Leave for a minimum of forty-eight hours before moving or attempting to use to ensure the blend hardens completely.

Lip Balm

1 ounce beeswax
1 ounce shea butter
2 ounces coconut oil
60 drops peppermint essential oil (you can substitute with lavender, sweet orange, lemon, grapefruit, lime)

On a stove in a double boiler with a glass insert, melt beeswax, and then, with a glass rod, stir in coconut oil. Once the coconut oil is melted, add shea butter and stir until completely melted. Remove from stove and add essential oil. Pour into lip balm tubes or tins. If you are using tubes, be sure to keep upright for at least two hours and do not use for at least forty-eight hours to ensure the blend has had time to cure.

Vanilla-Lavender Himalayan Salt Scrub

1 1/2 oz. finely ground Himalayan sea salt
1 T vanilla-infused jojoba wax
9 drops lavender essential oil

Using a two-ounce PET plastic jar, it fill with sea salt and oils. Stir the mixture using a glass stirring rod until all the ingredients are well mixed. Use caution in getting out of shower or bathtub, as the oils will make the surface slightly slippery.

Christine's Basic Bath Bomb Recipe

3 cups baking soda
1 1/2 cups citric acid
1 1/2 cups corn starch
3 T borax
Food grade coloring powder to your color preference
1 oz. mango butter
1 oz. cocoa butter
1.6 oz. grape seed oil
1/2 oz. distilled water
1/2 oz. clear alcohol
2 T essential oil of your choice

Mix all of the powders together in a stand mixer. On the stove, in a double boiler (with glass insert), melt all of the butters and oil and set it aside. Combine the water mixture with the oil mixture once butters have cooled to touch but are not completely cooled. With the mixer on low, pour liquids into dry mix. Increase the speed slightly—once. Once it is mixed well, turn the mixer back to low and mix for an additional two minutes. Test the mixture to make sure it holds its shape. Fill the molds with the mixture. Be sure to pack the mixture hard and firm into molds. Remove from the mold and allow it to dry and continue to harden for twenty-four hours.

Skin Toner

10 drops lavender essential oil
8 drops frankincense essential oil
6 drops geranium essential oil
4 drops German chamomile essential oil
1 oz. witch hazel
4 oz. distilled water

Mix all ingredients into a PET plastic or glass spray bottle. Be sure to shake well before each use to ensure the blend is well mixed. Use as a skin toner before your moisturizer each morning and evening.

Nourishing Body Oil

6 drops neroli essential oil
4 drops frankincense essential oil
2 drops lemon essential oil
1 oz. grape seed oil
1 oz. vanilla-infused jojoba wax

Mix the ingredients in a PET plastic or glass bottle. Use after bathing or any time your skin needs a little nourishing.

Dry Skin Moisturizing Oil

4 drops helychrysum essential oil
2 drops melissa essential oil
1 oz. avocado oil

Mix the ingredients in PET plastic or glass bottle. Use it on your skin in the evening before retiring to bed, and let this blend work on rejuvenating your skin through the night.

Spray-on Deodorant

5 drops sweet orange essential oil
3 drops lavender essential oil
2 drops frankincense essential oil
1 oz. witch hazel—alcohol free

Mix the ingredients in a PET plastic or glass spray bottle. Shake well before each use. Spray under armpits and let air dry

Passionate Body Spray

10 drops neroli essential oil
2 drops ylang ylang
2 drops frankincense
1 oz. distilled water

Mix the ingredients in a PET plastic or glass spray bottle. Shake well before each use. Spray on sheets, on pillows, and around the bedroom.

Clay Face Mask

1 tsp. kaolin clay
1 tsp. bentonite clay
2 drops myrrh essential oil
1 tsp. avocado oil

Mix the ingredients in a small bowl. Add avocado oil slowly to ensure a texture that is to your liking. Apply it gently to your face, avoiding the eyes, and let them dry for ten minutes. Wash your face with warm water, again avoiding the eyes. Pat dry with a towel.

Brown Sugar Scrub

5 oz. organic brown sugar
2 1/2 oz. vanilla infused jojoba wax
15 drops Myrrh essential oil
10 drops frankincense essential oil
4 drops lavender essential oil

In an eight-ounce PET plastic container, mix all the ingredients with a glass stirring rod until you reach a texture that is easily scoopable with your fingers. You can use additional jojoba to achieve the blend you desire. Use a small palm full while in the shower to help exfoliate. Use caution around your face. This mixture will make the shower floor slippery, so use caution when getting out of the shower/tub.

Minor Cuts and Scrapes

1 drop hylichrysum essential oil
1 drop lavender essential oil

Immediately after a minor cut or scrape, drop this combination on the site. It will help support minor bleeding control and aid in continued healing support.

Summer-Time Foam Soap

20 drops lemon essential oil
10 drops tea tree essential oil
45 ml castile soap

In a fifty-milliliter foam soap container, place essential the oil drops and then castile soap. Place a top on the container and give it a gentle shake. Lemon essential oil can be exchanged for a different essential oil depending on your aroma desire.

Hand Cleanser

20 drops lavender essential oil
15 drops lime essential oil
5 drops Tea Tree essential oil
2 oz. Aloe Vera Gel

In a two-ounce PET plastic, flip-top container, place the essential oil drops followed by aloe vera gel. Give it a gentle shake to mix the ingredients. Keep this mixture with you for times when you need a little hand cleansing and you do not have access to water. Be sure to gently shake the container before each use.

HOUSEHOLD AND CLEANING

Before you use any of the following blends on the surfaces in your home, be sure to check with the manufacturer to ensure that the surface is safe to have essential oils used on them for cleaning. Some surfaces are too delicate to have the oils used on them. If you have pets in your home, do not use any of these recipes on areas where your pets will walk. Pets like to lick their paws, and essential oils are not good for them to ingest, especially our feline fur family members who lack the proper enzymes to metabolize the oils. Expired essential oils are great to use for cleaning products.

Veggie Spray

1 cup apple cider vinegar
1 cup distilled water
10 drops tea tree essential oil
10 drops lemon essential oil

In a PET plastic or glass spray bottle, place essential oil drops followed by vinegar and water. Place spray top on and gently shake it to ensure a good mixture. Spray on the veggies when you bring them home from the store. Let the mixture sit for two to three minutes and then wash it off with warm, soapy water and dry. You will need to make a new batch every two to three weeks, as it has no preservatives in it.

Kitchen Counter Cleaner

1 cup white vinegar
1 cup distilled water
8 drops grapefruit essential oil
7 drops lime essential oil
5 drops tea tree essential oil

In a PET plastic or glass spray bottle, place the essential oil drops followed by vinegar and water. Place the spray top on and gently shake it to ensure a good mixture. Spray on the kitchen counter surface and wipe it clean with a soft cloth or paper towel. Be sure to gently shake it before each use as oils will separate. You will need to make it new every two to three weeks, as it has no preservatives in it.

Drain Freshener

1/2 cup baking soda
1/2 cup white vinegar
5 drops sweet orange essential oil
5 drops tea tree essential oil

Mix the ingredients and pour half of the mixture down each side of the sink. Allow it to sit for ten minutes and then rinse with soapy, warm water for five minutes.

Trash Can Freshener

1/2 cup baking soda
1/2 cup corn starch
1/4 cup Epsom salt
2 t water
10 drops lemon essential oil
10 drops sweet orange essential oil

In a glass bowl, combine the dry ingredients and mix well. Slowly add water and essential oils and stir it with a glass stirring rod until the mixture holds together when rolled into small balls. Using an ice cube tray, pack the mixture well into each square. Be sure not to overfill. Let it sit overnight and slowly remove it from the tray and place it in the bottom of the trash can. Replace as needed. Be sure to *not* use the ice cube tray for anything else other than making fresheners.

Awesome Oven Cleanser

1/2 cup salt
1/4 cup washing soda
2 cups baking soda
1/2 cup distilled water 1/4 cup white vinegar
1 T castile soap
10 drops lemon essential oil
10 drops sweet orange essential oil

Combine the ingredients in a glass bowl and form a spreadable paste. Apply it using latex gloves and a sponge and let sit for thirty to forty-five minutes. Wipe the oven clean with a cloth or sponge and water. You may need to wipe it down a few times to remove all residue.

Grill Cleanser

1/2 cup baking soda
3 T castile soap
5 drops lemon essential oil
5 drops tea tree essential oil
White vinegar

In a glass bowl, mix baking soda and castile soap with a glass stirring rod. Add essential oil drops, and mix. Add enough vinegar to make a runny paste. Remove the grill grate from the grill, and brush the mixture onto the entire grill grate. Let it sit for twenty to thirty minutes, wash it clean with soapy water, and rinse thoroughly. Dispose of the brush or label accordingly and use it only for this purpose in the future.

Sparkly Clean Window Cleaner

1 cup distilled water
2 tsp. white vinegar
2 tsp. alcohol
3 drops lemon essential oil

In a PET plastic or glass spray bottle, place essential oil drops followed by vinegar and water. Place the spray top on and gently shake it to ensure a good mixture. Spray on a window or mirror and wipe it clean with a soft cloth or paper towel. Be sure to gently shake it before each use as oils will separate. You will need to make it new every two to three weeks, as it has no preservatives in it.

Toilet Bowel Cleaner

1/2 cup baking soda
1/2 cup borax
1/4 cup white vinegar
10 drops lemon essential oil
10 drops tea tree essential oil

Mix the ingredients and add them to the toilet bowel. Allow it to sit for fifteen minutes and then scrub with a toilet brush and flush.

Bathroom Cleaning Spray

3 oz. distilled water
2 tsp. castile soap
1/8 tsp. white vinegar
5 drops eucalyptus essential oil
15 drops lemon essential oil
15 drops lime essential oil

In a four-ounce glass or PET plastic spray bottle, add all of the ingredients. Place the sprayer on bottle and gently shake it to mix thoroughly.

I Love Lemon Room Spray

4 oz. lemon hydrosol
70 drops lemon essential oil

In a glass spray bottle, mix the hydrosol and essential oil. Place the sprayer on the bottle and gently shake it to mix thoroughly. Spray a few sprays in any room to bring a fresh and renewed sense of energy to the room.

Yoga Mat Cleaning Spray

20 drops Tea Tree essential oil
15 drops peppermint essential oil
10 drops Eucalyptus
2 oz. lemon hydrosol

In a two-ounce glass or PET plastic spray bottle, add hydrosol up to neck of bottle (to leave room for essential oils). Place drops of essential oil to the bottle. Place the sprayer on the bottle and gently shake it until it is thoroughly mixed.

ROLLER BALL BLENDS

For these blends, we will be using ten-milliliter glass roller ball bottles. Roller balls can be used on pulse points or directly on areas of discomfort.

Sleep Well

3 drops neroli essential oil
3 drops lavender essential oil
2 drops frankincense essential oil
10 ml jojoba wax

Place essential oil drops into the roller ball container, and add jojoba wax. Place the roller ball on the bottle, snap it tight, and shake gently. Roll it behind the ears or on the temples twenty minutes before retiring for the evening.

Joint Ease

5 drops German chamomile essential oil
3 drops ginger essential oil
10 ml trauma oil

Place essential oil drops into the roller ball container, and add trauma oil. Place the roller ball on the bottle, snap it tight, and shake gently. Roll on areas of discomfort to help support easing painful joints.

Tense Away

6 drops marjoram essential oil
2 drops peppermint essential oil
10 ml trauma oil

Place essential oil drops into roller ball container, and add trauma oil. Place the roller ball on the bottle, snap it tight, and shake gently. Roll on areas of tension to help support relaxation of tense muscles in your body.

Tenacity

4 drops ravintsara essential oil
2 drops thyme linalol essential oil
2 drops laurel leaf essential oil
10 ml fractionated coconut oil

Place essential oil drops into a roller ball container, and add coconut oil. Place the roller ball on the bottle, snap it tightly, and shake gently.

Ahhhhh—Relaxation at Last

4 drops cypress essential oil
2 drops Roman chamomile essential oil
2 drops clary sage essential oil
10 ml fractionated coconut oil

Place essential oil drops into a roller ball container, and add coconut oil. Place the roller ball on the bottle, snap it tightly, and shake gently.

Sleepy Time

4 drops lavender essential oil
2 drops sandalwood essential oil
2 drops German chamomile essential oil
2 drops frankincense essential oil

Place essential oil drops into the roller ball container, and add coconut oil. Place the roller ball on the bottle, snap it tightly, and shake gently.

Immune Support

2 drops ravintsara essential oil
1 drop frankincense essential oil
2 drops lemon essential oil
1 drop lavender essential oil
1 drop vetiver essential oil
10 ml fractionated coconut oil

Place essential oil drops into the roller ball container, and add coconut oil. Place the roller ball on the bottle, snap it tightly, and shake gently.

Pick Me Up

3 drops lime essential oil
3 drops grapefruit essential oil
2 drops rosemary essential oil
10 ml fractionated coconut oil

Place essential oil drops into the roller ball container, and add coconut oil. Place the roller ball on the bottle, snap it tightly, and shake gently.

Serenity

2 drops ylang ylang essential oil
2 drops lavender essential oil
1 drop marjoram essential oil
1 drop sandalwood essential oil
1 drop neroli essential oil
10 ml fractionated coconut oil

Place essential oil drops into a roller ball container, and add coconut oil. Place the roller ball on the bottle, snap it tightly, and shake gently.

Let It Go

4 drops sweet orange essential oil
2 drops cardamom essential oil
1 drop juniper berry essential oil
1 drop myrrh essential oil
10 ml fractionated coconut oil

Place essential oil drops into a roller ball container, and add coconut oil. Place the roller ball on the bottle, snap it tightly, and shake it gently.

Get Fired Up

3 drops peppermint essential oil
3 drops ginger essential oil
2 drops sweet basil essential oil
10 ml fractionated coconut oil

Place essential oil drops into a roller ball container, and add coconut oil. Place the roller ball on the bottle, snap it tightly, and shake gently.

Shielded

4 drops geranium essential oil
2 drops juniper berry essential oil
2 drops black pepper essential oil
10 ml fractionated coconut oil

Place essential oil drops into a roller ball container, and add coconut oil.
Place the roller ball on the bottle, snap it tightly, and shake gently.

Changing It Up

4 drops lemongrass essential oil
2 drops cypress essential oil
2 drops elemi essential oil
10 ml fractionated coconut oil

Place essential oil drops into a roller ball container, and add coconut oil.
Place the roller ball on the bottle, snap it tightly, and shake gently.

DIFFUSER BLENDS

These blends are based on a hundred-milliliter diffuser reservoir. If your particular diffuser has a different size, please adjust the recipe accordingly.

Citrus Burst

3 drops tangerine essential oil
1 drop lemon essential oil
1 drop grapefruit essential oil

Fresh Floral

2 drops geranium essential oil
2 drops lavender essential oil
2 drops Roman chamomile

Spiced Cider

3 drops sweet orange essential oil
1 drop cinnamon essential oil
1 drop ginger essential oil

Summer Focus

3 drops eucalyptus essential oil
2 drops lime essential oil
1 drop rosemary essential oil

Joy in Your Morning

3 drops lemon essential oil
1 drop neroli essential oil
1 drop melissa essential oil

Stress Away

3 drops spike lavender
1 drop clary sage essential oil
1 drop sweet orange essential oil

Hot Flash Be Gone

3 drops peppermint essential oil
3 drops clary sage essential oil

Slim Down

4 drops grapefruit essential oil
2 drops cinnamon essential oil

Merry Christmas

3 drops cinnamon essential oil
2 drops sweet orange essential oil
1 drop clove bud essential oil

Peace Be with You

3 drops vetiver essential oil
2 drops frankincense essential oil
1 drop ylang ylang essential oil

Christine Stalsonburg

Remember This

3 drops rosemary essential oil
2 drops lime essential oil
1 drop peppermint essential oil

Pumpkin Pie

3 drops cardamom essential oil
1 drop sweet orange essential oil
1 drop cinnamon essential oil
1 drop clove bud essential oil

Energizer Bunny

3 drops lemon myrtle essential oil
2 drops grapefruit essential oil
1 drop Douglas fir essential oil

Meditate Me

3 drops neroli essential oil
1 drop opoponax essential oil
1 drop cedarwood essential oil

O Tannenbaum

3 drops scotch pine essential oil
2 drops Douglas fir essential oil
1 drop white pine essential oil

Warm Me Up

3 drops ginger essential oil
2 drops juniper berry essential oil
1 drop clove bud essential oil

Calm That Cough

3 drops cedarwood essential oil
2 drops larch tammarack essential oil
1 drop eucalyptus essential oil

Spice It Up

3 drops ginger essential oil
1 drop cardamom essential oil
1 drop black pepper essential oil

Three Wise Men

2 drops frankincense essential oil
2 drops myrrh essential oil
2 drops elemi essential oil

Protection

3 drops white angelica essential oil
2 drops frankincense essential oil
1 drop sweet orange essential oil

Joyfully Grounded

3 drops opoponax essential oil
1 drop marjoram essential oil
1 drop cedarwood essential oil

Hot Apple Cider

2 drops sweet orange essential oil
2 drops nutmeg essential oil
1 drop clove essential oil

Sweet Smell of Spring

3 drops lemon essential oil
2 drops jasmine essential oil

Peacetime

3 drops bergamot essential oil
2 drops palo santo essential oil
1 drop neroli essential oil

Festively Fall

3 drops cypress essential oil
2 drops sweet orange essential oil
1 drop vetiver essential oil

Autumn Morning

3 drops grapefruit essential oil
2 drops sweet basil essential oil
1 drop clove bud essential oil

Island Life

3 drops sweet orange essential oil
2 drops ginger essential oil
1 drop peppermint essential oil

Maui Magic

2 drops neroli essential oil
2 drops jasmine essential oil
2 drops sandalwood essential oil

Nana's Angel

3 drops white angelica essential oil
1 drop neroli essential oil
1 drop lavender essential oil

Kissed by the Sun

2 drops juniper berry essential oil
2 drops grapefruit essential oil
1 drop tangerine essential oil

Christine Stalsonburg

Mountain Lakes

3 drops lavender essential oil
2 drops sitka spruce essential oil
1 drop peppermint essential oil

Resources

The following are trusted resources that I have personally researched and used in making my own blends for my practice. They have shown, in my humble opinion, to be some of the best resources for your essential oil journey.

Essential Oils

Aromatics International, www.Aromatics.com

Bottles and Jars

SKS Bottles, www.sks-bottle.com

Carrier Oils

Aromatics International, www.Aromatics.com

Pink Himalayan Salt

Salt Works, www.Saltworks.com

Education and Training

Aromahead Institute, www.Aromahead.com

References

Battagli S. *The Complete Guide To Aromatherapy.* 2nd edition, 2003. The International Centre Of Holistic Aromatherapy.

Davis P. *Aromatherapy A-Z.* New revised edition. 1999. C.W. Daniel Company Limited.

International Federation of Professional Aromatherapists. *Pregnancy Guidelines.* www.itparoma.org, 2013.

Lawless J. *The Encyclopedia of Essential Oils.* 1995. Elemental Books Limited.

Majay G. *Aromatherapy For Healing The Spirit.* 1996, Henry Holt and Company Inc.

Tisserand, Robert and Young, Rodney. *Essential Oil Safety.* 2nd edition, 2014.

Tisserand, R. *The Art Of Aromatherapy.* 1977. Healing Arts Press

Zeck, Robbi. *The Blossoming Heart Aromatherapy For Healing and Transformation.* 2004 Aroma Tours

Acknowledgments

My journey with essential oils has been an amazing one. I have many people to thank for making me the aromatherapist I am today. Each and every one who has crossed my path in this journey has had an important part in the writing of this book.

First and foremost, my husband, Larry, has stood by me with love and support. He has believed in me and my goals to bring the knowledge in this book to the public. Through his encouragement, I was able to stay focused over the course of the eight months it took to write *Heaven Scent*.

Thanks to Andrea Butje, founder of Aromahead Institute, for her amazing abilities to bring education to aromatherapists. Her safe approach to using essential oils has awakened me to how I wanted to run my practice, Angelic Energy Massage Therapy and Wellness Center. I reference and use what I was taught by her daily, and for that I will be eternally grateful.

Thank you to Amy Hanson, my graphic designer, who has been a total joy to work with on this project. She gets me and my vision and brought that to life in the cover of *Heaven Scent*.

Thank you to my family and friends for believing in me and supporting me in this writing journey.

Thank you to God for giving me the gift to bring all of my education, experience, and passion together in a format that can be shared with others.

About the Author

Christine is a licensed massage therapist, certified aromatherapist, reiki master, angel therapy practitioner and owner of Angelic Energy Massage Therapy and Wellness Center. Through her years in practice, she has developed a gentle and safe approach to guiding her clients to total wellness through supporting the mind, body, and spirit.